EMDR Supervision

This unique handbook provides a guide for supervisors of therapists who use Eye Movement Desensitisation and Reprocessing (EMDR) therapy, and those undergoing training in EMDR supervision.

Whilst drawing on the literature on supervision theory and research, this book provides a down-to-earth guide to this topic, focusing on the European system of accreditation. The book guides the EMDR supervisor and supervisor-in-training in the difficult task of balancing the roles of educator, enabler, and evaluator.

Using the author's unique blend of warmth, humour, and humility, the book includes vignettes of real-life situations encountered by the author and provides practical solutions to dilemmas encountered in EMDR supervision.

Dr Robin Logie is a Clinical Psychologist and an EMDR Europe accredited Consultant and Trainer. He has taught on Consultants Trainings in the UK and Egypt and presented on EMDR supervision at conferences in the UK and Europe. He is on the accreditation committees for two national EMDR Associations.

T0384875

EMDR Supervision

A Handbook

Robin Logie

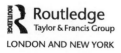
Routledge
Taylor & Francis Group

LONDON AND NEW YORK

Designed cover image: Alex Nail

First published 2024
by Routledge
4 Park Square, Milton Park, Abingdon, Oxon OX14 4RN

and by Routledge
605 Third Avenue, New York, NY 10158

Routledge is an imprint of the Taylor & Francis Group, an informa business

British Library Cataloguing-in-Publication Data
A catalogue record for this book is available from the British Library

ISBN: 978-1-032-10284-9 (hbk)
ISBN: 978-1-032-10283-2 (pbk)
ISBN: 978-1-003-21458-8 (ebk)

DOI: 10.4324/9781003214588

Typeset in Times New Roman
by MPS Limited, Dehradun

To Jane

Contents

Acknowledgements

I am indebted to the following colleagues and friends who have taken the time to look at earlier drafts of this book and share with me their valuable comments: Rachel Clarke, Omar Sattaur, Sandi Richman, Naomi Fisher, and Karen Beswick. Thanks also to Jo Scott and Marian Tobin for allowing me to reproduce their useful checklists in the Appendices.

Thank you to Alex Nail (my son-in-law), landscape photographer, who supplied the cover photo, taken at Langisjor in Iceland (www.alexnail.com).

As well as for her valuable comments on my book, I wish to thank my wife, Jane Logie, for her constant support and enthusiasm throughout the preparation of this book.

Introduction

For the last decade or so, I have been immersed in EMDR supervision and have become increasingly surprised that little has been written about this unique activity which is being practised by thousands of EMDR therapists and their supervisors across the world every day. "Well, I can't wait for someone else to write this book," I thought. "Perhaps I need to write it myself."

I am well aware that there exist hundreds of books on the topic of clinical supervision, both general and specific. "So why do we need one which is explicitly about EMDR supervision?" you may ask. Actually, the more that I have read about supervision generally and as it applies to other therapeutic modalities, the more I think, "yes, but that's not quite how we EMDR supervisors do it." For example, I have been astounded by how little exists in the literature on supervision regarding the "Supervision Question" which is a cornerstone of EMDR supervision and the way in which we train our EMDR Consultants.

Whilst all the relevant theory and accompanying references will be there, this volume should be seen very much as a "handbook" which will be like a Haynes Manual. These manuals were originally written for those who wanted to work on their own cars and I, myself, possessed such a manual as a young man in order to tinker with my first car, a Morris Minor Traveller (Haynes, 2012). Looking at their website as I write this, I see that Haynes' strapline "shows you how." Well, that is what I hope my book will do. My aim is to provide a handbook which is practical and "hands-on." If you are new to supervision and unfamiliar with the theory, you may want to read it from cover to cover. If you are an experienced supervisor and knowledgeable about supervision theory, you may be more interested in the more EMDR-specific aspects of the book. Experienced EMDR supervisors will want to dip in and out and have the book handy to guide them when they are having difficulties with supervision. And throughout this book I will be considering how things can go wrong during supervision and suggest ways of looking differently at what is occurring in the supervisory relationship, taking a step back, and thereby finding a new way forward.

DOI: 10.4324/9781003214588-1

There won't be illustrations and cross-sections of engines as you would find in a Haynes manual. But instead, there will be illustrations in the form of vignettes from my own experience and those of my colleagues. As a therapist, I have a particular interest in the value of storytelling as a therapeutic tool (Logie et al., 2020) and telling stories is very much how I teach my trainees and supervisees. So, this book will contain stories by way of illustrations. Many of these stories will be about the mistakes I have made, because we often learn more by hearing about mistakes than by getting things right.

Let me start by guiding you through the book and showing you what will be covered: The first chapter will start by asking "What is Supervision?" so that we can agree what we are talking about for the rest of the book. It will go on to discuss why supervision is necessary and look at the evidence that it actually makes a difference to our practice as therapists. The second chapter will examine what is different and unique about EMDR supervision. This chapter will provide the rationale for the whole book, because if there is nothing unique about EMDR supervision, this book would not be necessary.

In Chapter 3 we will look at ways of conceptualising EMDR supervision by drawing on existing supervision models. Do not skip this chapter, unless you already have an in-depth knowledge of supervision theory, because all subsequent chapters will refer constantly to the theory. One of the models outlined in this chapter, regarding the "formative," "restorative," and "normative" functions of supervision (which I have renamed "Educating," "Enabling," and "Evaluating"), then forms the basis for the next three chapters. The first of these is about educating and learning the EMDR protocol. The second is about enabling, supporting, and encouraging the therapist. The third is about evaluating the therapist's practice and ensuring that they are practising safely. A fourth chapter will be about how we need to balance these three complementary functions of supervision.

A further chapter will focus on Challenges in Supervision and will cover topics such as diversity, problems in the supervisory relationship, and how to manage unsatisfactory performance.

This takes us to Chapter 9 where I will consider how to provide EMDR supervision in groups and, in particular, a protocol that I have devised to really involve the group in the supervision process. Chapter 10 examines the mechanics of supervision and the advantages and disadvantages of providing supervision in different modalities. This chapter also looks at the different media in which the supervisee's practice can be observed. In Chapter 11 we look at a specific type of supervision which is the live supervision by facilitators at EMDR trainings. In Chapter 12 I will describe the ways in which we train EMDR therapists to become Consultants and how to evaluate EMDR supervisors.

Finally, it should be noted that, whilst attempting to pitch this book at an international audience, I am hampered by the fact that I have practised, taught, and supervised EMDR therapy only in the United Kingdom.

Therefore, some readers may find the book to be rather UK-centric. However, the EMDR Association UK is closely allied to EMDR Europe whose standards we adhere to in relation to criteria for accreditation for EMDR Practitioners, Consultants, and Trainers. This book will therefore be particularly relevant to readers in Europe although it is hoped that much of it will also be relevant to readers from other parts of the world.

Haynes. (2012). *Morris Minor 1000 (56–71) Haynes Repair Manual.* Yeovil, UK: Haynes Publishing.
Logie, R., Bowers, M., Dent, A., Elliot, J., O'Connor, M., & Russell, A. (2020). *Using stories in EMDR. A guide to the storytelling (narrative) approach in EMDR therapy.* Brighton: UK: Trauma Aid UK.

Chapter 1

What is supervision?

- Defining "supervision"
- "Supervision" vs "Consultation"
- How does supervision differ from training?
- How does supervision differ from therapy?
- Does supervision actually improve the therapist's skills?
- Therapist retention, well-being, and resilience
- Does supervision affect the likelihood of EMDR being practised?

Defining "supervision"

Before proceeding any further with a book on clinical supervision, I need to define what is meant by the term "supervision." This is not as easy a task as it may seem because there appears to be nearly as many definitions of "supervision" as there are textbooks on the subject.

Rather than immediately homing in on a fixed definition of supervision for the purposes of this book, I will start by discussing concepts in relation to defining supervision before gradually moving towards a working definition. Perhaps a good way of starting is with the writing of Joyce Scaife. "However supervision is defined, and whatever it means to you and me, it can be regarded as one way of getting help with our work" (Scaife, 2019, p. 26).

It is useful to differentiate between the *purposes* of supervision and the *functions* of supervision. Generally, the *purpose* is the reason for doing something. The *functions* are the kind of actions necessary to achieve this purpose. Starting with the purposes of supervision, I am reminded of the outrageous comment made by the British TV presenter Ann Robinson on a programme about one's pet hates, entitled *Room 101*. The BBC received 447 complaints after Robinson said of the Welsh, "I've never taken to them. What are they *for*?" So, firstly what is supervision *for*? Carroll (1996) defined the primary purposes of supervision as ensuring the welfare of clients and enhancing the development of the supervisee in work. In order to put these into effect, the

DOI: 10.4324/9781003214588-2

functions of supervision are education, support, and evaluation. These functions have traditionally been described as "formative," "restorative," and "normative" since Inskipp and Proctor (1993) although I will return to these later in this book and suggest my own alternative descriptive terms.

I have discovered two contrasting definitions of supervision which I find to be useful. The first, by Derek Milne (2007), is very specific and operational and is what I like to describe as the "bones" of supervision. The second, by Joyce Scaife (2019), gives me more of a feel of what supervision is actually like and is what I refer to as the "flesh" of supervision.

Derek Milne, coming from the British CBT perspective, has probably invested more energy than anyone else in attempting to clearly identify how to define clinical supervision. Milne (2007) conducted a systematic review in order to develop an empirical definition of clinical supervision. This included drawing meaningful boundaries between supervision and other closely related concepts such as "therapy," "coaching," or "mentoring," as well as a definition from which can be derived valid hypotheses and has been supported by empirical research.

In its most basic form, Milne's definition reads thus:

'FORM' OF SUPERVISION:
'The formal provision by senior/qualified health practitioners of an intensive relationship-based education and training that is case-focused and which supports, directs and guides the work of colleagues (supervisees).'

'FUNCTIONS' OF SUPERVISION:

1 quality control
2 maintaining and facilitating the supervisees' competence and capability; and
3 helping supervisees' to work effectively

(Milne, 2007, p. 440)

Milne adds "clarifying comments" to elaborate this definition as follows:

'FORM' OF SUPERVISION:
'The formal provision (i.e. sanctioned by relevant organization/s); by senior/ qualified health practitioners (or similarly experienced staff) of an intensive (i.e. typically 1:1 and regular/ongoing, at least, three meetings with protected time, of at least 3 hours total duration), relationship-based (inc. confidential and highly collaborative, being founded on a learning alliance and featuring (e.g.) participative decision making and shared agenda setting; and therapeutic inter-personal qualities, such as empathy and warmth), education and training (general problem-solving capacity or 'capability' aspect, not just competence enhancement) that is case-focused (supervisee guides topics and tables material and supervisor typically overlays professional and organizational considerations/standards) and which supports, directs and

guides (inc. also 'restorative and normative' topics, addressed by means of professional methods, inc. objective monitoring, feedback and evaluation; and by reference to the empirical and theoretical knowledge-base) **the work of colleagues (supervisees)** (inc. CPD/post-qualification colleagues)

'FUNCTIONS' OF SUPERVISION:
1   **quality control** (inc. 'gatekeeping' and safe, ethical practice);
2   **maintaining and facilitating the supervisees' competence and capability; and**
3   **helping supervisees' to work effectively** (inc. promoting quality control and preserving client safety; accepting responsibility and mostly working independently; developing own professional identity; enhancing self-awareness and resilience/effective personal coping with the job; critical reflection and lifelong learning skills).

(Milne, 2007, p. 440)

And now on to the "flesh" of supervision. Rather than provide a fixed definition of clinical supervision, Scaife (2019) suggests a list of aspirations for what clinical supervision should be, adapted from the characteristics of clinical supervision described by Cutcliffe and Lowe (2005). This list is also used by Sandi Richman when teaching EMDR Consultants Trainings in the UK:

Clinical supervision:

- Is supportive
- Takes place is the context of a facilitative relationship
- Is centred on developing best practices for service users
- Is challenging
- Is brave (because practitioners are encouraged to talk about the realities of their practice)
- Is safe (because of clear, negotiated agreements by all parties with regard to the extent and limits of confidentiality)
- Provides an opportunity to ventilate emotions without comeback
- Is not to be confused or amalgamated with managerial supervision
- Provides the opportunity to deal with material and issues that practitioners may have been carrying for many years (the chance to talk about issues which cannot easily be talked about elsewhere and which may have been previously unexplored)
- Is not to be confused or amalgamated with personal therapy or counselling
- Offers a chance to talk about difficult areas of work in an environment where the other person attempts to understand
- Is regular
- Takes place in protected time
- Is offered equally to all practitioners

- Involves a committed relationship from both parties
- Is an invitation to be self-monitoring
- Can be both hard work and enjoyable
- Is concerned with learning to be reflective and with becoming a reflective practitioner
- Is an activity that continues throughout one's healthcare career

(Scaife, 2019, pp. 31–32)

To me, this reads almost like a poem at times. It is not a clear definition but leaves one with a sense of what clinical supervision should be about. It should be noted however that Scaife omits to mention the Evaluating (or "normative") function of supervision which Milne describes as "quality control."

"Supervision" vs "consultation"

It is particularly important, especially in relation to the international readership of this book, that I make it clear what is meant by the word "supervision" and how it relates to the term "consultation." Unfortunately, these terms carry different meanings in Europe as compared to North America.

In North America the terms "supervision" and "consultation" have quite distinct meanings as explained by Bernard and Goodyear (2019), the most definitive text on supervision in the United States:

Supervision and consultations are very similar processes ... but supervisors have two responsibilities that consultants do not: They are responsible for the well-being of the clients their supervisees are treating; and they are responsible for ensuring that the supervisees have the necessary competence to move to a next level of training or responsibility.

(Bernard & Goodyear, 2019, p. 11)

To clarify this distinction, specifically in relation to EMDR supervision/consultation, I am quoting here from an article (Madere et al., 2020) published in the *Journal of EMDR Practice and Research* regarding "consultation" in the Eye Movement Desensitization and Reprocessing International Association (EMDRIA) that monitors standards in North America and is the organisation equivalent to EMDR Europe:

For purposes of this article, "supervisor" refers to a senior clinician who provides a pre-licensed psychotherapy (or provisionally licensed) clinician with oversight as required by state law, and holds legal responsibility for services provided by the supervisee. Secondarily, a licensing board may require a licensee to obtain supervision for a period pursuant to an administrative settlement of a formal complaint. In this second role, the supervisor is generally not legally responsible for the services provided by the supervisee, but is required to *evaluate* the nature, scope, and manner in which the supervisee provides psychotherapy services according to administrative requirements. In either case, a supervisor may or may not offer expertise in a therapy model such as EMDR.

In contrast, a consultant is providing peer consultation (EMDRIA, 2000), within a collaborative relationship (EMDRIA, 2019), from a position of more experience with regard to EMDR therapy. Obtaining consultation from a more senior clinician is common in the field of psychotherapy. In many regulatory and professional association guidelines, licensees are ethically obligated to seek such consultation regularly. It is the assumption of the authors that the consultant (or CIT) *is not* also the current supervisor of the consultee, as these roles are different and distinct. Nonetheless, throughout the consultation relationship consultants may discover the limitations of their consultees in much the same way that supervisors do with supervisees (American Counseling Association, 2014). Identifiable instances that a regulatory board or a court of law may find a consultant responsible include (a) if a board /court can show where/ how a consultant influenced the choices of consultees' work with a client using clear directives; and (b) if the board/court can show that the consultant knows the identity of the client(s).

(Madere et al., 2020, p. 6)

Because this book is being written from a European perspective, I am using the term "supervision" in the broadest sense, as it is used in Europe, to refer to all forms of supervision and consultation, not just in the narrower sense in which this term is employed in North America. Generally, as EMDR supervisors, we do not have clinical or legal responsibility for our supervisees' clients. We do have a responsibility, however, to report to our supervisee's employer and/or accrediting body if we have serious concerns about their practice which cannot be addressed in supervision. This will be covered in Chapter 8.

It should be noted however, that for some supervisees, the role of the supervisor will also involve responsibility for the supervisee's clients if, for example, the supervisee is a clinical psychologist in training and their EMDR supervisor is also their placement supervisor.

How does supervision differ from training?

In EMDR therapy there is a clear link between training and supervision. In fact, built into our current basic training in EMDR therapy, the supervision of cases is included from the Part 2 training onwards. In addition, the EMDR training includes live supervision during the training whilst trainees practise EMDR themselves during the training. We should therefore be clear how "supervision" differs from "training."

Training is "structured education for groups of trainees … [and] involves a standardized set of steps" (Hill & Knox, 2013, p. 776). This is elaborated upon by Bernard and Goodyear (2019) who state that, "whereas teaching is driven by a set curriculum or protocols, supervision is driven by the needs of the particular supervisee and his or her clients" (p. 10). In EMDR supervision we will often be doing some teaching, perhaps on a specific aspect of the Standard Protocol which was covered in the supervisee's training. But, in this case, the teaching will be tailored to the needs of the individual supervisee, and we may, for example, teach in such a way as is specific to that supervisee's own learning style and pre-existing knowledge.

Whilst the focus of this book is on supervision rather than training, it will also cover aspects of supervision (live supervision and supervision of cases) which actually occur during the course of the basic EMDR training.

How does supervision differ from therapy?

The more that I read and understand about the process of clinical supervision, the more I notice the parallels between what occurs in supervision and what occurs in therapy. So, before we tease out the ways in which they differ, let us first look at the ways in which supervision and therapy are similar.

This topic was covered in a seminal paper by Bordin (1983) who describes "an intimate connection between how one construes psychotherapy and how one construes supervision" (p. 35). Bordin describes the therapeutic relationship as a "working alliance," which is both "personal and technical" (p. 37). In supervision, the relationship between the supervisee and supervisor is as important as the technical and theoretical knowledge that the supervisor may impart. Without a relationship built on mutual trust, the supervisee will not disclose information about their clients in order to put themselves in a position to learn from their supervisor. Page and Wosket (2013) describe the similarities thus: "Two or more people come together, identify their respective roles and endeavour to assist those in the consumer role, whether clients or supervisees, with difficulties they bring to that setting. This is done using a range of interpersonal and therapeutic skills … being able to listen, hear, empathise, reflect, form and maintain a healthy and appropriate relationship, support, challenge, make connections, and intervene at a level appropriate to the recipient. All this takes place within agreed boundaries of time, place, regularity, confidentiality and payment" (p. 18). A particular way in which supervision appears to mimic therapy is through the phenomenon of the "parallel process" (Friedlander, Siegel, & Brenock, 1989) (to be covered in more depth later in this book) in which the dynamics of the therapy room are being re-enacted in the supervision room.

So, let us now be clear about the ways in which supervision *differs* from therapy. "In supervision, it is the therapy that is the 'patient' and the supervisee's feelings and fantasies are examined only insofar as they may throw light on what is happening in the therapy" (Mollon, 1989, p. 121). Page and Wosket (2013) differentiate supervision and therapy as follows.

Table 1.1 The differences between therapy and supervision
(simplified version of table in Page and Wosket, 2013)

	Therapy	Supervision
Aims	To improve the client's life.	To develop the supervisee's skills as a therapist.
Presentation	Client presents information verbally.	Supervisee presents through a variety of media.
Timing	Client may choose the pace.	Supervisee focuses on what needs to be covered to work effectively with their clients.
Relationship	The client is held emotionally and can regress and act out emotions.	The supervisory relationship is professional and collaborative.
Expectations	Client is not expected to prepare for the session.	Supervisee is expected to come prepared and with necessary materials.
Responsibilities	Therapist's responsibility is to the client.	The supervisor's responsibility to the client can take precedence over their responsibility to their supervisee.

However, there is an important difference between therapy and supervision that is not included in Page and Wosket's list. Beinart (2004) points out that supervision is primarily an educative process which involves the evaluation of the supervisee.

Finally, I need to address the issue of how supervision may, at times, tip into therapy without either party being aware of what is happening. Whilst Frawley-O'Dea and Sarnat (2001) observed that attempting "a rigidly impenetrable boundary between teaching and 'treating' in supervision is neither desirable nor truly achievable" (p. 137) there are boundaries that must not be crossed in supervision. Any therapeutic intervention should be limited to assisting the supervisee to work more effectively with the client under discussion and to go beyond this could be considered as ethical misconduct (Bernard & Goodyear, 2019).

This can be a delicate path to tread. A supervisee of mine was repeatedly telling me that, although she had a good grasp of the protocol, she was very anxious about commencing processing for fear of harming her client. She was aware that this was connected to earlier experiences, and it was something she needed to work on. She was actually meeting with someone, with whom she had done her EMDR training, for mutual EMDR sessions and agreed that she would take it there. Although I did not provide her with any therapy, I did make some suggestions as to what to target in the therapy.

Does supervision actually improve the therapist's skills?

In a longitudinal study (Goldberg et al., 2016), clinical outcomes were measured for 170 therapists with up to 18 years' experience. Outcomes did not increase with experience and, if anything, they deteriorated slightly. The study does not state the extent to which the therapists were receiving supervision, but it does highlight the fact the experience alone is not enough to make you an effective therapist.

Thinking specifically about EMDR therapy, we have a clear protocol and there is evidence that adhering to the protocol achieves better therapeutic outcomes. Farrell and Keenan (2013) found that EMDR therapists who had achieved accreditation were generally reporting better outcomes from EMDR therapy than those who had not been accredited. This offers some evidence that EMDR supervision may improve treatment outcomes although it has to be accepted that accredited therapists are also likely to be more invested in EMDR being effective. However, this finding is confirmed by the study by Maxfield and Hyer (2002) which found a correlation between treatment fidelity and clinical outcomes with EMDR.

I have to confess at this point to my own "wilderness years" as I like to call them. After completing my basic EMDR training in 1997, I did not receive any EMDR supervision until 2005. I was finding EMDR to be effective and was happy with my practice. But when I did start receiving supervision, I realised that I had drifted quite radically from the Standard Protocol. I was, in fact, quite astonished, when looking back at my original training manual, that I was doing things quite differently from what I had been taught on my basic EMDR training. My supervisor successfully whipped me into shape, and I started using EMDR in a more incisive and effective way. Since then, I have realised the importance of continued supervision.

One published study specifically examines the extent to which clinical supervision can directly increase treatment fidelity with an evidence-based therapy. Bearman et al. (2017) looked at the effectiveness of clinical supervision upon clinicians trained in CBT:

> Specifically, those who received supervision that included skill modeling, role-play, and corrective feedback based on session review showed a pattern of incremental improvement across the three supervision meetings on cognitive restructuring fidelity, CBT expertise, and global CBT competence. These participants were rated as proficient or near proficient on all three outcomes by the final assessment.
>
> (Bearman et al., 2017, p. 12)

In contrast, the participants whose supervision did not include these specific components did not improve following the assessment that occurred immediately post-training. Other studies have also supported these findings (Martino et al., 2016; Webster-Stratton, Reid, & Marsenich, 2014).

Obviously treatment fidelity is a specific issue for the practice of EMDR therapy (Madere et al., 2020). There is some empirical evidence that supervision enhances adherence to a particular manualised procedure (e.g. Hildebrand et al., 2012).

What is the research evidence that clinical supervision enhances client outcomes? A great deal of research has been carried out in this area and, in a review of reviews, Watkins (2020) stated that the evidence is still very unclear. He concluded that supervision is positively associated with job satisfaction, job retention, and ability to manage workload. It is seen as helpful by supervisees and may even benefit their therapeutic competence. But supervision's impact on actual client outcome is not so clear. "Scholarly opinion – based upon the supposed weight of empirical evidence – is that supervision contributes to supervisee competence development and skill transfer, but any impact on client outcome has yet to be proven" (Watkins, 2020, p. 14). These were broadly the same results of a review by Tugendrajch et al. (2021) who concluded that supervision enhances therapist self-efficacy, therapist competence, and therapist alliance with their clients but there is no clear effect on actual client therapeutic outcomes. A meta-analysis by Whipple et al. (2020) is less optimistic, concluding that the amount of variance in client outcome attributable to clinical supervision was less than 1%. In reviewing the literature in this area, Hawkins and McMahon (2020) conclude:

> There are indications that for supervision to contribute to positive outcomes, it may need to be regular and frequent, include structure rather than just support, and be focussed on specific therapeutic skills or therapeutic alliance development. It also appears that these factors may be particularly important for benefiting the clients of trainees, those learning new therapeutic models, and those navigating new work contexts. (p. 270)

Most of what they state appears to be particularly relevant, specifically in relation to EMDR supervision.

Therapist retention, well-being, and resilience

After the somewhat disappointing evidence from the previous section, let us look, finally, at the importance of clinical supervision for retention, well-being, and resilience. This is what one of my supervisees has written about the supervision that they have received:

> I have found the supervision invaluable. I have found it helpful to work through cases in which I feel I have become a bit stuck or where I have not been sure which route to take. The supervision has also helped with increasing my confidence in my approach and with following my intuition. I have found it helpful how you talk about your own mistakes, or when things haven't gone according to plan, as this helps me with feeling able to accept my own mistakes and to not put too much pressure on myself to have

to get it 'right' all the time. I also value the examples that you share of your own experience when your approach has worked well and when you are able to tell me when you don't know the answer (which is quite reassuring).

Supervision is an essential "professional watering hole" (Grant & Schofield, 2007, p. 11) and was named as one of the top three sources of professional development (along with client experience and personal therapy) amongst therapists in the USA (Norcross, 2005). In a review of 21 studies with USA child welfare practitioners, whilst the evidence base for the effectiveness of supervision was found to be "weak," they found that organisational commitment to supervision and having supportive supervisors were associated with professionals' decisions to remain in the workplace. Supervision was also related to job satisfaction. One study has shown that supervision reduces burnout and stress (Wallbank, 2013) whilst another showed its value in improving staff well-being and productivity (Hyrkäs, Lehti, & Paunonen-Ilmonen, 2001).

So, whilst the jury may still be out in relation to the evidence that effective supervision may result in better client outcomes, it is clearly regarded as a valuable activity amongst therapy professionals.

Does supervision affect the likelihood of EMDR being practised?

My own clear anecdotal evidence, as an EMDR trainer, is that trainees are very unlikely to start practising EMDR in their place of work if they are not in receipt of EMDR supervision. There is evidence to support this finding (Dodaj & Dodaj, 2021; Grimmett & Galvin, 2015; Kerr, 2009). This will be covered in more depth in Chapter 5 but it is important to make this point here in order to support supervision as an activity.

Conclusion

The purpose of this chapter has been to set the scene for the rest of the book. We need to have a clear understanding as to what supervision actually means and how it differs from other activities in our work such as therapy and teaching. Most importantly this chapter has outlined why supervision is such a valuable and important practice for all EMDR therapists.

American Counseling Association. (2014). *ACA code of ethics*. Alexandria, VA.

Bearman, S. K., Schneiderman, R. L., & Zoloth, E. (2017). Building an evidence base for effective supervision practices: An analogue experiment of supervision to increase EBT fidelity. *Administration and Policy in Mental Health and Mental Health Services Research, 44*(2), 293–307.

Beinart, H. (2004). Models of supervision and the supervisory relationship. In I. Fleming & L. Steen (Eds.), *Supervision and clinical psychology* (pp. 47–62). Hove, East Sussex: Routledge.

Bernard, J. M., & Goodyear, R. K. (2019). *Fundimentals of clinical supervision* (6th ed.). New York, NY: Pearson.

Bordin, E. S. (1983). A working alliance based model of supervision. *The Counseling Psychologist, 11*(1), 35–42.

Carroll, M. (1996). *Counselling supervision: Theory, skills and practice*. London: Cassell.

Cutcliffe, J. R., & Lowe, L. (2005). A comparison of North American and European conceptualizations of clinical supervision. *Issues in Mental Health Nursing, 26*(5), 475–488.

Dodaj, A., & Dodaj, A. (2021). Experience of an EMDR practitioner in EMDR education: Case report. *Psychiatria Danubina, 33*(Suppl 1), 100–102.

EMDRIA. (2000). *EMDRIA consultation packet*. Austin, TX: EMDR International Association Online Community.

EMDRIA. (2019). *EMDRIA consultation packet*. Austin, TX: EMDR International Association Online Community.

Farrell, D., & Keenan, P. (2013). Participants' experiences of EMDR training in the United Kingdom and Ireland. *Journal of EMDR Practice and Research, 7*(1), 2–16.

Frawley-O'Dea, M. G., & Sarnat, J. E. (2001). *The supervisory relationship: A contemporary psychodynamic approach*. New York: Guilford Press.

Friedlander, M. L., Siegel, S. M., & Brenock, K. (1989). Parallel processes in counseling and supervision: A case study. *Journal of Counseling Psychology, 36*(2), 149.

Goldberg, S. B., Rousmaniere, T., Miller, S. D., Whipple, J., Nielsen, S. L., Hoyt, W. T., & Wampold, B. E. (2016). Do psychotherapists improve with time and experience? A longitudinal analysis of outcomes in a clinical setting. *Journal of Counseling Psychology, 63*(1), 1.

Grant, J., & Schofield, M. (2007). Career-long supervision: Patterns and perspectives. *Counselling and Psychotherapy Research, 7*(1), 3–11.

Grimmett, J., & Galvin, M. (2015). Clinician experiences with EMDR: Factors influencing continued use. *Journal of EMDR Practice and Research, 9*(1), 3–16.

Hawkins, P., & McMahon, A. (2020). *Supervision in the helping professions* (5th ed.). London: Open University Press.

Hildebrand, M. W., Host, H. H., Binder, E. F., Carpenter, B., Freedland, K. E., Morrow-Howell, N., ...Lenze, E. J. (2012). Measuring treatment fidelity in a rehabilitation intervention study. *American Journal of Physical Medicine & Rehabilitation, 91*(8), 715–724.

Hill, C., & Knox, S. (2013). Training and supervision in psychotherapy. In M. Lambert (Ed.), *Bergin and Garfield's handbook of psychotherapy and behavior change*, 6th ed (pp. 775–811). New York: Wiley.

Hyrkäs, K., Lehti, K., & Paunonen-Ilmonen, M. (2001). Cost–benefit analysis of team supervision: the development of an innovative model and its application as a case study in one Finnish university hospital. *Journal of Nursing Management, 9*(5), 259–268.

Inskipp, F., & Proctor, B. (1993). *The art, craft and tasks of counselling supervision. Part 1-making the most of supervision*. 4 Ducks Walk, Twickenham, Middlesex: Cascade.

Kerr, C. (2009). *Why do some EMDR trained therapists choose not to integrate this therapy into their practice to work with PTSD?* (MSc thesis), University of Chester.

Leeds, A. (2016). *A guide to the standard EMDR protocols for clinicians, supervisors and consultants* (2nd ed.). New York: Springer.

Madere, J., Leeds, A., Sells, C., Sperling, C., & Browning, M. (2020). Consultation for EMDRIA certification in EMDR: Best practices and challenges. *Journal of EMDR Practice and Research, 14*, 1–14.

Martino, S., Paris Jr, M., Añez, L., Nich, C., Canning-Ball, M., Hunkele, K., ...Carroll, K. M. (2016). The effectiveness and cost of clinical supervision for motivational interviewing: a randomized controlled trial. *Journal of Substance Abuse Treatment, 68*, 11–23.

Maxfield, L., & Hyer, L. (2002). The relationship between efficacy and methodology in studies investigating EMDR treatment of PTSD. *Journal of Clinical Psychology, 58*(1), 23–41.

Milne, D. (2007). An empirical definition of clinical supervision. *British Journal of Clinical Psychology, 46*(4), 437–447.

Mollon, P. (1989). Anxiety, supervision and a space for thinking: Some narcissistic perils for clinical psychologists in learning psychotherapy. *British Journal of Medical Psychology, 62*(2), 113–122.

Norcross, J. C. (2005). The psychotherapist's own psychotherapy: Educating and developing psychologists. *American Psychologist, 60*(8), 840.

Page, S., & Wosket, V. (2013). *Supervising the counsellor: A cyclical model.* London: Routledge.

Scaife, J. (2019). *Supervision in clinical practice: A practitioner's guide* (3rd ed.). Milton Park, Abingdon, Oxon: Routledge.

Tugendrajch, S. K., Sheerin, K. M., Andrews, J. H., Reimers, R., Marriott, B. R., Cho, E., & Hawley, K. M. (2021). What is the evidence for supervision best practices? *The Clinical Supervisor, 40*(1), 68–87.

Wallbank, S. (2013). Maintaining professional resilience through group restorative supervision. *Community Practitioner, 86*(8), 26–28.

Watkins Jr, C. E. (2020). What do clinical supervision research reviews tell us? Surveying the last 25 years. *Counselling and Psychotherapy Research, 20*(2), 190–208.

Webster-Stratton, C. H., Reid, M. J., & Marsenich, L. (2014). Improving therapist fidelity during implementation of evidence-based practices: Incredible years program. *Psychiatric Services, 65*(6), 789–795.

Whipple, J., Hoyt, T., Rousmaniere, T., Swift, J., Pedersen, T., & Worthen, V. (2020). Supervisor variance in psychotherapy outcome in routine practice: A replication. *SAGE Open, 10*(1), 1–11, 2158244019899047.

What is different and unique about EMDR supervision?

- Is there an EMDR supervision model?
- Integrating EMDR with an existing therapeutic modality
- Can we assume that EMDR trainees possess the basic skills required before starting their EMDR training?
- Integrating supervision with basic training
- The Supervision Question
- Teaching from the theory
- Contracting
- Keeping records of supervisees

Indeed, what is the point of this book? There are many excellent books published on the topic of clinical supervision. So, if there was nothing unique about EMDR supervision, there would be no need for this book. In this chapter, I demonstrate what is unique and different about EMDR supervision and the justification for a book such as this.

Is there an EMDR supervision model?

I will try to answer this question by using an analogy from within our own work as EMDR therapists. As most readers will know, in the EMDR world there is a tendency amongst some EMDR therapists to clamour for a specific protocol for each separate psychological disorder. For example, "what is the EMDR protocol for OCD?" There are, indeed, several published protocols for OCD (Logie, 2019). "So, which is the best and which one should I use for my client?" The answer may be that we need to obtain a thorough history before producing a clear case conceptualisation using the AIP model and then the course of action may become obvious to us. The protocols that we have read about in relation to OCD may then inform us about how to apply the AIP model to your particular client. But slavish adherence to a particular protocol without really understanding what is going on for your client is unlikely to be helpful and could be counterproductive.

DOI: 10.4324/9781003214588-3

The same applies, in my opinion, with regard to seeking a specific EMDR supervision model. Like the specific protocols for OCD, there may be particular considerations in relation to EMDR supervision which set it apart from supervision for other therapeutic modalities and it is these differences that I will be addressing in this chapter. But essentially EMDR supervision and the supervisory relationship will bear a remarkable similarity to the way in which supervision occurs in other modalities.

There has been a tendency for each therapeutic modality to produce their own way of conducting supervision by drawing on their own model of providing therapy. So, for example, CBT supervision will include agenda setting, Socratic questioning and homework which are, of course, all elements of a CBT therapy session (Corrie & Lane, 2015; Milne, 2018). By contrast, psychodynamic supervision is more supervisee-centred and gives greater attention to the supervisee's own dynamics (Ekstein & Wallerstein, 1958).

In a study by Putney et al. (1992), CBT supervisors were perceived to be in a consultant role and to focus on skills and strategies more than were humanistic, psychodynamic, and existential supervisors, who were perceived more as using the relationship model, playing the therapist role, and focusing on conceptualisation. Supervisors were not perceived to differ in their use of growth and skill development models, teacher roles, and focus on the supervisee.

It is interesting to note, however, that even CBT supervision draws upon therapies derived from other therapeutic modalities and, in particular, psychodynamic theories. For example, the Seven-Eyed Model (see Chapter 3) (Hawkins, 1985) which looks at supervision in a relational and systemic way, is often cited in texts relating to CBT supervision (e.g. Milne, 2018).

There is an argument moreover that using a therapy model to understand what is happening in supervision is unhelpful. Supervision differs from therapy in that it is fundamentally a reflexive process within which an educational element is an important part to facilitate the learning of professional skills and roles (Beinart & Clohessy, 2017) as I outlined in Chapter 1. It has also been argued that the use of therapy models to explain the learning process may hinder professional development and may lead to boundary infringement between supervision and therapy (Ladany, 2014). Milne (2018) points out that we need to be clear about how our supervision model differs from the therapy model.

So, to what extent should EMDR supervision draw upon our own Adaptive Information Processing (AIP) model (Shapiro, 2007)? At first sight, the AIP model does not immediately lend itself to a clear way of doing supervision. One of the things that initially attracted me to EMDR was that, in my opinion, it draws on the "best bits" of several older therapeutic modalities. The AIP model itself shares with psychodynamic psychotherapy and Trauma-focused CBT, for example, the idea that we need to go back to the experience of the original trauma in order to process it. From mindfulness approaches comes the instruction to "just notice," from psychodynamic therapy comes free association, from body therapies come the link with the felt sense in the body, and from CBT comes the structured aspects of the Assessment Phase. So, it is my contention that, in a similar way, our model of supervision should take the "best bits" from the ways in which these other therapies are supervised (Hawkins & McMahon, 2020). So looking again at the study by Putney et al. (1992) (see above) I would hope that EMDR supervision focuses on skills and strategies but also focuses on case conceptualisation and the supervisory relationship.

What follows is my understanding as to what is unique and different about EMDR supervision.

Integrating EMDR with an existing therapeutic modality

The first unique aspect of EMDR supervision, which I will discuss, relates to the fact that, with a few exceptions, EMDR trainees are already trained and experienced in another therapeutic modality before training in EMDR therapy. Let us illustrate this with what Naomi Fisher, EMDR Consultant, said to a group of her supervisees who were all new to EMDR therapy:

> When people start learning EMDR they can feel really de-skilled. It feels like, "Errh! This new thing I've got to learn how to do." But actually, you keep all of your other skills and EMDR, you can integrate it and all the systemic thinking and everything, it's all still completely relevant. You're still highly skilled professionals who are learning a new skill which will integrate and then you'll be, like, amazing!

> People often think, "oh, I don't know what to do now", and it's almost like they forget everything else and they think, "I've got to do this new thing. I've got to follow the protocol."

One of the roles of the EMDR supervisor is to assist the therapist in integrating what they already know into the AIP model and a new way of working as an EMDR therapist. Hawkins and McMahon (2020) explain that one of the aspects of learning a new way of conceptualising one's work is the "unlearning" of old ways of thinking. "Unlearning involves recognising our habitual patterns and often unaware ways of doing things and interrupting them to provide the space to begin new approaches" (p. 20). But, perhaps it is something different to "unlearning" that our trainees need to achieve. As Naomi demonstrated above, it is about integrating something new with what you already know. At an online workshop regarding EMDR supervision in 2020, Derek Farrell referred to the concept of "pattern matching" in which trainees attempt to understand new concepts regarding EMDR by comparing them with what they already understand about their existing way of conceptualising their work (Farrell, 2020). Come to think of it, this is, in fact, the AIP process in action where we attempt to assimilate new experiences into our pre-existing under-standing of ourselves and the world. In a study by Dunne and Farrell (2011), 45% of EMDR trainees reported a difficulty incorporating EMDR into their practice due to their pre-existing therapeutic modality. This was a particular issue for those previously trained in analytic and humanistic therapies. (I will return to this issue in more depth in Chapter 4 in which I discuss the teaching of the AIP model and EMDR Standard Protocol.)

None of this makes EMDR supervision different to other forms of super-vision *per se*. However, it means that the EMDR supervisor has an additional task which is not always present in supervision for other therapeutic modalities.

Can we assume that EMDR trainees possess the basic skills required before starting their EMDR training?

The obvious answer to this question is "no!"

Each national EMDR association produces a set of criteria related to professional groups and clinical experience which must be satisfied by can-didates prior to acceptance on basic EMDR training courses. It is my view that these groups are selected on the basis that they possess the following basic skills:

• Understanding of *psychological theory*
• *Case formulation*
• Forming a *therapeutic relationship*
• Following a *manualised approach*
• Understanding the *system* in which the therapy takes place

I will now explain each of these in more detail.

Understanding of psychological theory

In order to produce a case formulation for a particular client (discussed next) the therapist needs a basic background in psychological theory. Particularly relevant theories are likely to be attachment theory and learning theory. In addition, for individuals working with children and adolescents, an under-standing of developmental psychology is essential.

Case formulation

This connects closely to the understanding of psychological theory but is a distinct skill which involves applying psychological theory to the understanding of particular individuals who come for therapy. These skills will be developed during actual training as a therapist and will largely be honed through the clinical supervision that the therapist receives whilst on placement.

Perhaps a distinction should be made between diagnostic skills and case formulation skills. The former relates to the classification of individual clients according to diagnostic categories such as obsessive-compulsive disorder (OCD). However, I contend that the AIP model demands that we understand our client's current symptoms not in terms of what is wrong with them but in terms of what has happened to them (Johnstone et al., 2018).

Forming a therapeutic relationship

EMDR therapy occurs in the context of a therapeutic relationship. The client needs to feel that they can trust their therapist and vice versa. EMDR is a powerful therapy and can involve intense abreaction at times. The therapist needs to have the ability to "hold" the client at these times and for the client to feel safe and held (Dworkin, 2013).

Following a manualised approach

In my trainings, I have noticed that some very experienced and insightful therapists who can form a good therapeutic relationship, may really struggle with the EMDR protocol and, in particular, the Assessment Phase. They are not familiar with following instructions from a manual or worksheet and find that this conflicts with their usual way of relating to their clients.

Understanding the system in which the therapy takes place

Not always, but often, it is the context of the client's problems that are important to understand in order to provide effective therapy. This is the case particularly when working with children; whichever therapy is utilised, the family system and educational system may need to be taken into account.

In my experience as an EMDR supervisor, it is often our role to assist our supervisees with the inevitable gaps in their pre-existing skills as they become apparent. I can think of a particularly promising supervisee who had previously trained as a counsellor and had a real feel of how to do EMDR. However, his understanding of psychological therapy and case conceptualisation meant that he needed more help than most in target selection and on occasions I would need to stop and explain, for example, some aspects of Attachment Theory with which he was unfamiliar. In contrast, another supervisee understood the mechanics of EMDR very well and had few problems in proceeding correctly through the Standard Protocol. But on viewing her video I became aware that the way in which she related to her client was not conducive to a trusting and secure therapeutic relationship.

Integrating supervision with basic training

The model of EMDR training used in Europe integrates supervision and training from the very start. During the Part 1 training, clinicians start to practise EMDR therapy with each other, receiving live supervision as they do so (see Chapter 11). As soon as trainees have completed their Part 1 training, they are expected to start using EMDR with their clients and to receive regular supervision in their place of work as well as, subsequently, on the further parts of their basic training. After the basic training ends, therapists are encouraged to start the process of working towards Practitioner accreditation under guidance from their supervisor and this is considered to be the next stage in their training to become a competent EMDR therapist.

EMDR therefore differs from some other therapeutic approaches in that the supervision is an integral part of the training. Whilst the supervision they receive will, in many respects, be no different to the type of supervision they might receive for another therapy, an element of the supervision received is an essential extension to their basic training. In my experience, there are always gaps in what my supervisees have recalled or learnt from their basic training, and I believe it is the responsibility of the supervisor to find these gaps and plug them!

The Supervision Question

As well as "teaching from the theory," one of the first things trainee EMDR Consultants learn in their training is the importance of the Supervision Question. This may not be something they have encountered before in previous supervision training or in the therapeutic modality in which they were previously working.

The concept of the "Supervision Question" is not unique to EMDR. However, I have been surprised that there is very little mention of this important method in the literature on clinical supervision. Under a section entitled, "Creative Approaches," one of the most respected texts on supervision (Scaife, 2019) says, "they can quickly reach the heart of the matter [by asking the] supervisee … to identify her or his dilemma with the client in a single sentence" (p. 228). Padesky (1996) describes starting a supervision session with "informational questions" (Padesky, 1993) such as "how can I help your today?" or "how would you prioritize your concerns?" On her website (Padesky, 2014), Christine Padesky states that "my ground rules for supervision include: Always ask a supervision question before saying anything about the case. Try to be specific and avoid general questions like, 'What should I do with this client?'" Beinart and Clohessy (2017) say, "some supervisors expect a supervisee to bring a prepared supervision question to help focus the session so that they can make the best use of the time available" (p. 77). Gordon (2012) says that the Supervision Question

gives clarity about the goal of the ensuing discussion, it ensures the work stays on track (with the implied test of 'Have we answered the question?')

and as Bordin (1983) has pointed out, it promotes an active stance in the supervisee and strengthens the working alliance (p. 73).

So why do we pay particular attention to the Supervision Question in EMDR supervision? It is time for another analogy: In EMDR therapy we often struggle with our clients to help them find their Negative Cognition (NC). This process will sometimes be quite lengthy, but it can be time well spent and the actual process of identifying the NC itself can be an important part of the therapy. On occasions, the client's discovery of their NC is a crucial turning point in the therapy before the actual Desensitisation Phase has even started. And so it is with the Supervision Question.

Often my supervisees are irritated by my insistence on them providing a Supervision Question. They just want to tell me about their client! But the Supervision Question provides the focus that I need as a supervisor to really help my supervisee to get what they want out of the session. It also helps me to know when to interrupt if I think that the information that they are providing is irrelevant to the Supervision Question.

Knowing what the Supervision Question is often alerts the supervisor to the fact that the supervisee may, in fact, be asking the "wrong" question. I will return to this in more detail in Chapter 7, but at this stage, it is important to point out that the supervisee's question may, for example, be in relation to what they are doing with their client and the fact that processing is not changing the SUDS scores. What they might really need to be asking, however, is a question regarding the formulation and an understanding as to what is actually going on with their client which might lead them to a different target memory.

Teaching from the theory

Another thing that we impress upon trainee EMDR Consultants is to "teach from the theory." This may seem obvious but is not something that is self-evident from reading the literature on clinical supervision.

As a supervisor, our instinct may often be to rescue our supervisee by telling them exactly what to do with a particular client. It reminds me of that old proverb: "Give a man a fish and you feed him for a day. Teach a man to fish and you feed him for a lifetime." By going back to some basic principles regarding EMDR, grounded in the AIP model, our supervisees will learn something, not just about how to work with this particular client, but how they may assist many other clients that they may encounter in the future.

Contracting

Osborn and Davis (1996) see the development of the supervision contract as a necessary ritual for both parties in the supervision process and doing so is an essential part of any clinical supervision endeavour regardless of the therapeutic modality. However, there are some unique characteristics in relation to how we would go about doing this as EMDR supervisors.

Sometimes, there is a rush for both the supervisee and their supervisor to start discussing cases before it is clear how they will be working together (Beinart & Clohessy, 2017). (Compare this with the EMDR therapist who rushes into the Desensitisation phase without adequate History Taking, case conceptualisation and Preparation.)

The first question to consider is whether the supervision will be uniquely in relation to just the practice of EMDR or whether it will cover the supervisee's clinical practice generally. I knew of an EMDR Consultant who said that his supervision would be just in relation to EMDR practice only and, if the supervisee had any other issues in relation to their therapy practice, they should take them elsewhere. As I will explain more fully in subsequent chapters, sometimes the reason why EMDR is not working may be because the therapist needs to take account of other non-EMDR-related factors. If this is the case, to limit EMDR supervision to only EMDR-related issues may be very restrictive. However, it should also be accepted that EMDR supervision should always have EMDR therapy as its focus and only move beyond EMDR when there is a good reason to do so. In any event, the initial contracting process should make this clear and it is important with a new supervisee to check whether they are receiving supervision elsewhere and what the nature of that supervision is. It should be clear whether the EMDR supervisor is also expected to be the therapist's generic supervisor and if so, whether there are legal and/or ethical issues to consider. For some core professions, there is a requirement that they also receive generic supervision from a member of their own professional group in order to maintain their accreditation.

For various reasons, some therapists will have more than one EMDR supervisor and this was my own situation for several years. As much as is possible I avoided discussing the same client with both supervisors as this would be confusing for me and also lead to an unnecessary degree of competition between the two supervisors.

The contract should set the scene for evaluation. In particular, will the supervisee be working towards accreditation? This is particularly relevant in EMDR supervision because it means that the supervisor would expect the supervisee to video their treatment sessions or allow the supervisor to sit in on such sessions. The contract itself should set the scene for the evaluation that will be an integral part of the supervision process (Bernard & Goodyear, 2019). The process of contracting will also help the supervisor to uncover what may be the supervisee's motivation for seeking supervision. This could be one or more of the following:

- The therapist seeks to enhance their clinical skills and improve as an EMDR therapist. If this is their only goal, they may have no interest in accreditation and be reluctant to present their work for evaluation.

- The therapist only wants supervision in order to become accredited. If this is the case, they may be reluctant to accept feedback from the supervisor and show little eagerness to learn. They may even cease supervision as soon as they become accredited.
- The therapist wants to "cover their back" in case any complaints are made about them and have no interest in either becoming accredited or learning to become a better EMDR therapist.

A thorough contracting process will help to make it clear which of these is motivating the therapist to come for supervision.

It should be accepted that contracting (rather like the History Taking phase of EMDR therapy) may be an ongoing process which one may need to return to at a later stage after several supervision sessions. "I find that contracting is usefully thought of as a process that occurs over a number of sessions, regularly or irregularly, and from time to time for the duration of the supervisory relationship" (Scaife, 2019, p. 59). For example, one of my supervisees initially approached me for supervision when I was a trainee Consultant and said it was fine because she had no plans to become accredited herself. As soon as I became an EMDR Consultant, she said that maybe she *would* like to work towards accreditation. Very soon she was accredited and went on to be the first person with whom I worked towards Consultant accreditation before a very fruitful career as an EMDR Consultant herself with many supervisees.

See Appendix 1 which shows an example of an EMDR supervision contract devised by Jo Scott. See also Appendix 2 devised by Marian Tobin with a checklist of things to ask a supervisee when starting supervision.

Keeping records of supervision

As an EMDR supervisor, you will need to consider carefully how you will record what occurs in each supervision session. This should be linked with the process of contracting, to accreditation and also the possibility that a complaint is made about your supervisee. Some of the things to consider are as follows:

- How will you take notes and where will your notes be stored (e.g. on paper, digitally, as part of the organisation's computerised recording system)?
- How can you record which clients and how many clients you have discussed with your supervisee for the purposes of accreditation?
- Will the notes be in the form of a supervision log?
- Will you be sharing your notes with your supervisee?
- How might your notes be used if a complaint is made about your supervisee?

Conclusion

Whilst EMDR supervision bears many similarities to clinical supervision in other therapeutic modalities, this chapter has outlined several distinct differences. Firstly, it occurs in the context of having supervisees who are already trained and experienced in other therapies and therefore this has to be taken into account in terms of how we help our supervisees make this integration. EMDR supervision is focused around the Supervision Question. This relates to adherence to the Standard Protocol of EMDR and should always be linked with the theory and, in particular, the AIP model. It is also closely integrated with the system by which EMDR therapists are trained. Contracting is a process in which this way of working can be made explicit and can be reviewed when necessary.

Beinart, H., & Clohessy, S. (2017). *Effective supervisory relationships. Best evidence and practice.* Chichester, UK: Wiley.

Bernard, J. M., & Goodyear, R. K. (2019). *Fundimentals of clinical supervision* (6th ed.). New York, NY: Pearson.

Bordin, E. S. (1983). A working alliance based model of supervision. *The Counseling Psychologist, 11*(1), 35–42.

Corrie, S., & Lane, D. (2015). *CBT supervision.* London: Sage.

Dunne, T., & Farrell, D. (2011). An investigation into clinicians' experiences of integrating EMDR into their clinical practice. *Journal of EMDR Practice and Research, 5*(4), 177–188.

Dworkin, M. (2013). *EMDR and the relational imperative: The therapeutic relationship in EMDR treatment.* London: Routledge.

Ekstein, R., & Wallerstein, R. S. (1958). The teaching and learning of psychotherapy (2nd ed.). New York, NY: International Universities Press.

Farrell, D. (2020). Advanced clinical supervision and consultation skills in enhancing competency in EMDR therapy. EMDR Lebanon Association

Gordon, P. (2012). Ten steps to cognitive behavioural supervision. *The Cognitive Behaviour Therapist, 5*(4), 71–82.

Hawkins, P. (1985). Humanistic psychotherapy supervision: A conceptual framework. *Self & Society, 13*(2), 69–76.

Hawkins, P., & McMahon, A. (2020). *Supervision in the helping professions* (5th ed.). London: Open University Press.

Johnstone, L., Boyle, M., Cromby, J., Dillon, J., Harper, D., Kinderman, P., …Read, J. (2018). *The power threat meaning framework: Towards the identification of patterns in emotional distress, unusual experiences and troubled or troubling behaviour, as an alternative to functional psychiatric diagnosis.* Leicester: British Psychological Society.

Ladany, N. (2014). The ingredients of supervisor failure. *Journal of Clinical Psychology, 70*(11), 1094–1103.

Logie, R. (2019). How does the literature inform us regarding the use of EMDR for the treatment of obsessive-compulsive disorder (OCD)? *EMDR Therapy Quarterly, 1*, 23–28.

Milne, D. (2018). *Evidence-based CBT supervision: Principles and practice* (2nd ed.). Hoboken, NJ: Wiley.

Osborn, C. J., & Davis, T. E. (1996). The supervision contract: Making it perfectly clear. *The Clinical Supervisor, 14*(2), 121–134.

Padesky, C. (1993). *Socratic questioning: Changing minds or guiding discovery.* Paper presented at the A keynote address delivered at the European Congress of Behavioural and Cognitive Therapies, London.

Padesky, C. (1996). Developing cognitive therapist competency: Teaching and supervision models. In P. Salkovskis (Ed.), *Frontiers of cognitive therapy* (pp. 266–292). New York: The Guilford Press.

Padesky, C. (2014). *Better supervision.* Retrieved from www.padesky.com/making-supervision-better

Putney, M. W., Worthington, E. L., & McCullough, M. E. (1992). Effects of supervisor and supervisee theoretical orientation and supervisor-supervisee matching on interns' perceptions of supervision. *Journal of Counseling Psychology, 39*(2), 258.

Scaife, J. (2019). *Supervision in clinical practice: A practitioner's guide* (3rd ed.). Milton Park, Abingdon, Oxon: Routledge.

Shapiro, F. (2007). EMDR, adaptive information processing, and case conceptualization. *Journal of EMDR Practice and Research, 1*(2), 68–87.

Chapter 3

Ways of understanding and conceptualising EMDR supervision

- Functions of supervision – the three Es – Educating, Enabling, and Evaluating
- Modes of supervision – The Seven-Eyed model
- Levels of supervision – "Developmental" models
- General Supervision Framework

Firstly, please do not skip this chapter! Much of what follows in subsequent chapters are based upon the theory outlined here and, if you do skip the chapter, you will only have to return to it later to make sense of what you have been reading. You have been warned!

This is not intended to be a comprehensive review of what has been written about the theory of supervision generally, since excellent such reviews already exist elsewhere (Bernard & Goodyear, 2019; Hawkins & McMahon, 2020; Scaife, 2019). Instead, I plan to review the literature on the theory of clinical supervision with direct reference to EMDR supervision. There has been a proliferation of published models of clinical supervision. A recent review (Simpson-Southward, Waller, & Hardy, 2017) identified 52 different models. I am following the sage advice of Bernard and Goodyear (2019): "If a model does not add clarity to the process for you, it could be that you simply think too differently from its author(s) for it to be useful. It is OK to reject a model for this reason. Models are created to be helpful resources to the supervisor, not intellectual burdens" (p. 69). I have therefore decided to refer only to those models of supervision that have a particular resonance for me in making sense of what is happening during EMDR supervision.

After reviewing the literature in relation to theories regarding clinical supervision (Logie, 2021), it appears to me that there are three main theoretical models of supervision which are particularly relevant and useful in understanding EMDR supervision. This also accords broadly with the conclusions of Farrell et al. (2013) in their paper on EMDR supervision. I describe these three models as being the "functions," "modes," and "levels" of supervision:

DOI: 10.4324/9781003214588-4

- The three *functions* of supervision (usually known as "formative," "restorative," and "normative"), the three Es – Educating, Enabling, and Evaluating
- The seven *modes* of supervision (the "Seven-Eyed" model)
- The four *levels* of supervision ("Developmental" models)

I will describe each of these in turn and explain how they are relevant to EMDR supervision.

Functions of supervision – The three Es – Educating, Enabling, and Evaluating

The terms "formative," "restorative," and "normative" were coined by Proctor (1988). However, prior to that, Kadushin (1976) used the words "educative," "supportive," and "managerial" for the same three functions and other authors such as Hawkins and Smith (2013) have used different terms for the same functions. "Formative," "restorative," and "normative" are most often used to describe these three functions amongst therapists, but not necessarily because they are the best words to describe them. I believe that they have stuck, perhaps, merely because they rhyme with each other! I would suggest alternative terms which I believe might be more appropriate in relation to EMDR supervision, namely "Educating," "Enabling," and "Evaluating." Initially, I called the first of these, "teaching" but a wise trainee on my Consultants Training pointed out that "educating" is more appropriate as it is more all-encompassing. In addition, she pointed out that, "Educating" starts with the letter "E" which means that all three functions can start with the same letter!

This is summarised in Table 3.1.

Table 3.1 Different terms for the three basic functions of supervision

Kadushin (1976)	Proctor (1988)	Hawkins and Smith (2013)	Logie
Educative	Formative	Developmental	Educating
Supportive	Restorative	Resourcing	Enabling
Managerial	Normative	Qualitative	Evaluating

The Educating function

For much of the time, what is occurring during a supervision session is educating. The supervisor may be teaching the therapist about the EMDR Standard Protocol or other EMDR protocols and how they may be relevant to the client under discussion. The supervisor may be helping the therapist to understand how their prior training in other modalities can be relevant to EMDR or how they need to case conceptualise. The supervisor may start by asking the therapist questions about the particular client and the therapist will be presenting information about the client and what work s/he has been doing with the client. The object of this will be for the supervisor to ascertain where the therapist may be going wrong or what gaps there may be in their knowledge, in order to assist the therapist to work more effectively with the client. During this time, the therapist will be learning something new about EMDR or about how to work more effectively as a therapist.

The Enabling function

Most supervisors will have supervisees who have a clear formulation in relation to their client and clearly understand the protocol and how it should be applied. But they are just not going ahead with EMDR or they are doubting their own ability or their client's readiness, for example, to commence processing. In such instances, what is required is not educating, but *enabling*. Here, it is the job of the supervisor to address the therapist's concerns and fears in relation to the work they are doing. We may not be teaching, so much as boosting our therapist's confidence. "That's great! Yeah, just crack on!" Sometimes, when the therapist seems really stuck, I ask the Flashforward (Logie & De Jongh, 2014) question: "what's the worst thing that could happen if you started processing now?" But sometimes the enabling function is more in relation to "sharing the awfulness," for example, when the therapist says, "I'm not stuck with this client, but I have just had a really upsetting session with them and I feel that I need to share it."

The Evaluating function

As an EMDR supervisor, our role is also to evaluate our supervisee's practice, particularly in relation to the process of accreditation. In this situation, we are neither educating nor enabling, but evaluating. There may be times during supervision when this is occurring in quite a formal way such as when we are viewing the supervisee's videos. But it is also likely to happen throughout the supervision process as we are gauging how well the supervisee is managing case conceptualisation or how well they appear to understand the Standard Protocol.

Note that the next three chapters will be addressing each of these functions in turn and discussing them in more depth.

Modes of supervision – The seven-eyed model

This story is about my own experience of being a supervisee many years ago, before I was involved with EMDR. I had a supervisor named Michael who is German and with whom I had an excellent supervisory relationship. I had an adolescent client, probably autistic, who repeatedly expressed neo-Nazi opinions during his sessions with me, making comments such as "six million Jews wasn't enough." As the son of a Jewish refugee from Nazi Germany myself, I was understandably very distressed by this and decided to take it to supervision although this was with some trepidation as I was aware that this might be difficult for Michael considering his own background. In supervision, I started by explaining the context of my distress by disclosing my own heritage which I had not previously done. Before we actually discussed my case, Michael disclosed that his wife was also from a Second-Generation German Jewish refugee family. He was very supportive and helpful in discussing this particular case. In fact, my wife and I later became friends with them both.

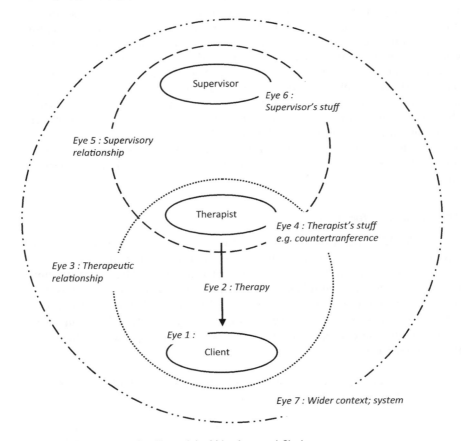

Figure 3.1 The "Seven-Eyed" model of Hawkins and Shohet

This story illustrates how what is happening with the client can have resonances for the therapist which, in turn, may affect the therapist/client relationship. When brought to supervision, the therapist's "stuff" may resonate with what is happening for the supervisor and bring up their own stuff which may, in turn, affect the supervisory relationship.

The easiest way to describe this model in diagrammatic form is as shown in Figure 3.1.

According to the Seven-Eyed model of supervision of Hawkins and Shohet (Hawkins, 1985; Hawkins & McMahon, 2020) the supervision process is seen through the lens of seven different "eyes," based on the three people to whom supervision relates:

- Supervisor
- Therapist (supervisee)
- Client

I will describe each of the seven "eyes" and how this may be relevant, in particular, to EMDR supervision.

Eye 1: The client

Often, what is occurring during a supervision session is that the therapist is describing the client, for example, the client's presenting problems, history, personal resources, or demeanour during the session. At this time, we are in Eye 1.

Eye 2: The therapy

Here, the therapist is describing to their supervisor or discussing with their supervisor what therapy they are providing, or they are contemplating what intervention they might take. The focus is on "what to do" i.e. the therapeutic intervention.

Eye 3: The therapeutic relationship

With this eye, the focus is not on the client or the therapy, but on the relationship between the client and therapist. At times, there may be problems in the therapy, not because the therapist does not understand the client (Eye 1) and not because they do not know an effective way of helping them (Eye 2) but because the therapeutic relationship is not conducive to therapeutic change. This may be due to lack of trust. It may be due to transference. The client may not want to "get better" because they might risk losing the relationship they have with their therapist.

Eye 4: The therapist's "stuff"

It may be that the therapist's own issues or unprocessed adverse life events are getting in the way of the therapy progressing. For example, the client reminds the therapist of their own mother or their client's experience of bereavement awakens unprocessed grief in the therapist. At times, supervision may need to address the therapist's difficulties that are triggered by what is happening in the therapy session. In EMDR therapy, we talk about the "blocking beliefs" held by the client which may impede processing in a therapy session. Similarly, the therapist may hold a blocking belief of their own which may prevent them from responding or acting in a way that is therapeutic to their client.

Eye 5: The supervisory relationship

Here the focus is on the relationship between the supervisor and therapist. There may exist tension between the supervisor and supervisee which bears no relation to the client in question. For example, the supervisee may be eager to be approved for accreditation by the supervisor and therefore fail to disclose their own doubts and mistakes in order to create a good impression.

However, the client under discussion might also affect what is happening in supervision. A "parallel process" (Doehrman, 1976; McNeill & Worthen, 1989) may be occurring in which the supervisory relationship is manifesting similar relationship dynamics to those in the therapeutic relationship. For example, a particular client may be very dependent on the therapist which may be reflected in the therapist appearing to be equally dependent on the supervisor when discussing this particular client. Or a client whose NC is "I'm not good enough" may manifest in the parallel process as the therapist feeling "I'm not a good enough therapist." What happens in the therapy room may be re-enacted in supervision (Bernard & Goodyear, 2019) and, conversely, what happens in supervision may be re-enacted in the therapy room (Frawley-O'Dea & Sarnat, 2001).

Eye 6: The supervisor's "stuff"

It may be that the supervisor's own unprocessed past experiences are getting in the way of them being able to effectively assist the therapist. This may be in the form of countertransference where the therapist reminds the supervisor of someone from the past with whom they had a difficult relationship that was never resolved.

However, it can also be useful for the supervisor to use their own emotional reactions as a barometer to ascertain what is occurring in the therapy room (Piedfort-Marin, 2021; Searles, 1955).

Eye 7: The system

Therapy always occurs in a context. For example, who is funding the therapy and what influence do they have about how it proceeds? If the therapy is on the National Health Service (NHS), is there a limit to the number of sessions or a limit on what events can be targeted during processing? If it is funded by a compensation claim, must the processing only be in relation to the accident in question? And if a relative is paying for the therapy, what is their attitude to the therapy and how it should be conducted? In this situation, the supervision is not related to three people (client, therapist, and supervisor) but to four or more.

Levels of supervision – "Developmental" models

A number of theories of supervision can be grouped into what are described as "developmental" models (Holloway, 1987). These describe the level the trainee has reached in terms of their development as a therapist and how this is relevant to how they are supervised.

The Integrated Developmental Model (IDM) of Stoltenberg and colleagues (Stoltenberg & McNeill, 2011; Stoltenberg, McNeill, & Delworth, 1988) is the best-known and most widely used developmental model of supervision.

Stoltenberg describes four stages (levels) of supervisee development within three overriding structures: The first of these structures is "self and other awareness," reflecting the level of the therapist's self-pre-occupation, self-awareness and awareness of the client's world. Secondly, "motivation" describes the therapist's interest, investment, and effort expended in clinical training and practice. The third structure is "autonomy" which describes the extent to which the therapist becomes independent. The four levels are as follows.

Level 1: Dependency stage

The supervisee experiences anxiety and insecurity whilst being highly motivated in the work. Awareness is self-focussed and performance anxiety is likely to be dominant. The therapist may be focusing mostly on surviving the session with the client. Because they are preoccupied with the rules, skills, theories, and didactic material being learned, the therapist may find it hard to tune into the process information that the client is providing. At this stage, the supervisor's job may be to provide safety and containment. Dependency and insecurity can manifest itself in different ways in the supervisory relationship. Some supervisees may cope with this situation by presenting as helpless, which forces the supervisor into the role of rescuer. Others may conversely present themselves as super-confident, saying that they understand everything, making it equally hard for the supervisor to assist them in supervision.

Level 2: Dependency-autonomy

At this stage, the supervisee fluctuates between feeling over-confident and feeling overwhelmed. (On some days I think I am still stuck at this stage myself!) The focus on supervision will move away from the supervisee themselves to the client. Therapists at this stage are still unlikely to be aware of countertransference issues that arise during therapy. At this stage, the supervisor needs to continue providing a "secure base."

Level 3: Conditional dependency

Therapists are developing increased self-confidence, greater insight and more consistency in their therapy sessions. They are more able to focus on the process. Supervision should be undertaken in a framework of enquiry in order to facilitate the development of self-supervision and reflective practice.

Level 4: Master professional

The therapist has personal autonomy, insightful awareness and can confront personal and professional issues themselves. The supervisory process becomes increasingly collegial, and the structure and process of the supervision session is more often determined by the therapist. Often the therapist will now be supervising others and supervision may involve discussion of issues with supervisees rather than clients, i.e. supervision of supervision or "metasupervision."

It should be accepted that these stages refer to a therapist's general development, not just in relation to a particular therapeutic modality such as EMDR. So, some of the issues, especially in relation to the earlier levels, may not apply to experienced and accomplished therapists who are new to EMDR. But even for such therapists, thinking about their level of development as an EMDR therapist can be useful when providing supervision.

In any event, the developmental level of the therapist may be particularly relevant to EMDR supervision. This is because the form that the supervision will take will depend to a large extent on the supervisee's level of EMDR training and development. At one end of the spectrum, the therapist has just completed their Part 1 training. At the other end of the spectrum, the therapist is an experienced EMDR Consultant or Trainer.

So how do these correspond to the stages of development of an EMDR therapist? In their paper, Farrell et al. (2013) describe a different developmental model (Dreyfus, 2004) and how it corresponds to the development of an EMDR therapist. I will do the same in relation to Stoltenberg's four stages in the IDM model.

Level 1: Dependency stage for EMDR therapists

This will apply to the stage where therapists are still in the process of undergoing their basic 7–8 day training in EMDR. Supervision is provided as part of the training and should also be provided on a regular basis after Part 1 of the training. Prior to completing the training, therapists have not yet even been taught the full EMDR protocol and, even after training has been completed, their grasp of the Standard Protocol may be tenuous. Therefore, much of what the supervisor will be doing is to provide reassurance and often quite basic didactic teaching in relation to the Standard Protocol.

Level 2: Dependency-autonomy for EMDR therapists

This level will be reached at some point after the basic EMDR training has been completed and will occur during the early stages prior to the therapist being ready to apply for Practitioner accreditation. The therapist will still be learning the Standard Protocol but will be able to work more autonomously and reflect to a greater extent upon their work.

Level 3: Conditional dependency for EMDR therapists

This stage will be reached after the therapist has been accredited as a Practitioner and may be working toward becoming an accredited EMDR Consultant. They should now have the Standard Protocol firmly in their grasp and be only consulting their supervisor about particularly complex clients and learning some advanced protocols.

Level 4: Master professional for EMDR therapists

This stage would be reached after the therapist becomes an accredited EMDR Consultant. The therapist will still bring clients to supervision with whom they have particular problems. At this stage, "supervision of supervision" or "metasupervision" may occur as the therapist discusses difficulties that they are having with particular supervisees (see Chapter 12). It should be acknowledged that not every supervisee will want or be capable of reaching this stage.

Looking at the developmental levels of EMDR according to Stoltenberg's framework may be a useful start, but for the purposes of conceptualising the development of an EMDR therapist, I believe that it is also helpful to think of the following six stages:

1   Trainee
2   Working towards Practitioner accreditation
3   Working towards Consultant accreditation

4   Post Consultant
5   Facilitator
6   Trainer

Some of the time periods and functions at each of these stages are summarised in Table 3.2.

Table 3.2 Giving and receiving supervision at different levels of development as an EMDR
therapist

	Time period	Receiving supervision	Supervising others	Receiving metasupervision	Facilitating	Training
Training	Preferably less than a year	Yes				
Trained	1 year plus	Yes				
Accredited	3 years plus	Yes	Training to supervise	Yes		
Consultant		Yes	Yes	Yes		
Facilitator		Yes	Yes	Yes	Yes	
Trainer		Preferably	Yes	Preferably	Yes	Yes

As EMDR supervisors, we should always be cognisant of which stage our
supervisee is at and tailor their supervision accordingly.

Stoltenberg (1981) says that, at the first stage of development, "the
developing counsellor is quite concerned with rules of counselling at this
point and is searching for the right way to do things" (p. 61). This would
certainly apply to the supervision of EMDR trainees. Bordin (1974) points
out that, at this stage of their development the trainee should be able to
observe their supervisor doing the therapy. This occurs during EMDR
training where trainees observe videos and live demonstrations of EMDR
therapy.

A specific issue I touched on in the previous chapter was of integrating
EMDR with a previously learned model. In connection with this, we also
need to consider that two supervisees who are both still at the training stage
of EMDR may have contrasting backgrounds and experiences. They may in
fact be sitting next to each other on a basic EMDR training. Let me typify
them both as follows:

•   John is a 60-year-old psychodynamic psychotherapist with 35 years of
    experience as a therapist.
•   Aisha is a 25-year-old trainee clinical psychologist who has only been
    seeing clients for a couple of years and is still learning the basics of CBT on
    her training course.

Although they are both "learning the ropes" in relation to the basic EMDR protocol they will each face quite different challenges in doing so. For John, forming a therapeutic relationship and knowing how to respond to his client may be quite intuitive and he is likely to have the confidence that comes with his age and experience. But he may struggle to unlearn some of his well-established ways of working and struggle in particular with following a manualised approach. By contrast, Aisha will be quite familiar with learning new techniques and will have the flexibility to adapt to a new protocol. However, she lacks the experience of John and her quite understandable anxiety may impede her ability to learn. Their training needs as supervisees are likely to be quite different. So whilst a particular therapist may be at "level 1" in relation to their EMDR practice they might be at "level 4" in relation to other domains of practice (Stoltenberg et al., 2014).

Once the supervisee is an EMDR Consultant (or training to become one) supervision can take on an additional dimension which becomes part of the therapist's training as a supervisor themselves. To illustrate this, let us look at a rough transcript of what occurred during one of my supervision sessions with an EMDR therapist who has recently become an EMDR Consultant:

Supervisee (after discussing a particular case):	I no longer feel like a useless therapist. I have realised that mum is not responding because she has her own unresolved trauma rather than because I am ineffective.
Robin:	OK, so how did I help you with that?
Supervisee:	By pointing this out and saying how *you* would feel in the same situation.

So, as well as providing supervision in relation to particular cases with which they are struggling, my supervision will also include some reflection on what is actually occurring during this process. I will refer to this in more detail in Chapter 12 on the training of EMDR supervisors.

Finally, it should be noted that much of the literature on clinical supervision, particularly in North America, is actually referring only to "trainee supervision," in other words, someone who has not yet completed their basic professional training. Much of the supervision that is occurring in EMDR elsewhere in the world should be referred to as "practitioner supervision" (Page & Wosket, 2013).

General supervision framework

Finally, I wish to refer, briefly, to a fourth supervision theory, the General Supervision Framework (Scaife, 1993) which I have found to be helpful. I do not consider it to be one of the three central planks referred to above (functions, modes, and levels) in which I conceptualise supervision, but is does constitute an additional useful way of looking at what is happening in EMDR supervision. It looks at the three following areas:

- Supervisor role behaviour
- Supervision focus
- Supervision medium

It is the first of these, "supervisor role behaviour," which particularly interests me. As a supervisor we are likely, at any one time, to be enacting one of the three following roles with our supervisee:

- Inform–assess
- Enquire
- Listen–reflect

Inform–assess

This involves making observations and judgement of the supervisee's performance, offering critical comments and "telling" things to the supervisee.

Enquire

Rather than telling stuff to the supervisee, the supervisor is asking questions from a spirit of curiosity and exploration.

Listen–reflect

This involves attentive listening and reflection in order to highlight and fully explore the issues raised.

In EMDR supervision there is a time and place for each of these roles. Lizzio et al. (2005) refer to the contrast between "didactic" and "facilitative" styles by supervisors. In their study, a facilitative, rather than didactic, supervisory approach positively influenced supervisees' perceptions of the effectiveness of supervision. However, in EMDR supervision there are moments when we just need to do some straight teaching and, in fact, our supervisees may become irritated by our Socratic questioning and say (or *feel* like saying), "just blooming well tell me what I am doing wrong!"

Compare this with what occurs in EMDR therapy. Whilst processing is occurring spontaneously, we "stay out of the way" and "trust the process," somewhat like the listen–reflect style of supervision. However, if the processing becomes stuck we use a therapeutic interweave and, similarly, as when our supervisee just doesn't know or understand something, we may just need to tell them!

Conclusion

The purpose of this chapter has been to provide the basic framework for the rest of the book. By conceptualising what is happening in supervision in terms of functions, modes and levels we can get a handle on what is actually occurring between ourselves and our supervisees. In this way, we can begin to reflect on what is happening, both when supervision goes well but also when things become stuck in supervision.

Bernard, J. M., & Goodyear, R. K. (2019). *Fundimentals of clinical supervision* (6th ed.). New York, NY: Pearson.

Bordin, E. S. (1974). Reflections on preparation for psychological counseling. *The counselor's handbook*. New York: Intext Educational Publishers.

Doehrman, M. J. G. (1976). Parallel processes in supervision and psychotherapy. *Bulletin of the Meninger Clinic, 40*, 9–104.

Dreyfus, S. E. (2004). The five-stage model of adult skill acquisition. *Bulletin of Science, Technology & Society, 24*(3), 177–181.

Farrell, D., Keenan, P., Knibbs, L., & Jones, T. (2013). Enhancing EMDR clinical supervision through the utilisation of an EMDR process model of supervision and an EMDR personal development action plan. *Social Sciences Directory, 2*(5), 6–25.

Frawley-O'Dea, M. G., & Sarnat, J. E. (2001). *The supervisory relationship: A contemporary psychodynamic approach*. New York: Guilford Press.

Hawkins, P. (1985). Humanistic psychotherapy supervision: A conceptual framework. *Self & Society, 13*(2), 69–76.

Hawkins, P., & McMahon, A. (2020). *Supervision in the helping professions* (5th ed.). London: Open University Press.

Hawkins, P., & Smith, N. (2013). *Coaching, mentoring and organizational consultancy: Supervision and development* (2nd ed.). Maidenhead: Open University Press.

Holloway, E. L. (1987). Developmental models of supervision: Is it development? *Professional Psychology: Research and Practice, 18*(3), 209.

Kadushin, A. (1976). *Supervision in social work*. New York: Columbia University Press.

Lizzio, A., Stokes, L., & Wilson, K. (2005). Approaches to learning in professional supervision: Supervisee perceptions of processes and outcome. *Studies in Continuing Education, 27*(3), 239–256.

Logie, R. (2021). Using supervision theory to enhance effective EMDR supervision. In R. Logie (Ed.), *EMDR Consultants Resources Book* (2nd ed.). Brighton, UK: Trauma Aid UK.

Logie, R., & De Jongh, A. (2014). The "Flashforward procedure": Confronting the catastrophe. *Journal of EMDR Practice and Research, 8*(1), 25–32.

McNeill, B. W., & Worthen, V. (1989). The parallel process in psychotherapy supervision. *Professional Psychology: Research and Practice, 20*(5), 329.

Page, S., & Wosket, V. (2013). *Supervising the counsellor: A cyclical model*. London: Routledge.

Piedfort-Marin, O. (2021). *The client-therapist relationship in EMDR psychotherapy. How to address these issues in consultation.* Paper presented at the EMDR Association UK. Consultants Day, London.

Proctor, B. (1988). Supervision: A co-operative exercise in accountability. In M. Marken, & M. Payne (Eds.), *Enabling and ensuring.* Leicester: National Youth Bureau and Council for Education and Training in Youth and Community Work.

Scaife, J. (1993). Application of a general supervision framework: Creating a context of co-operation. *Educational and Child Psychology, 10*(2), 61–72.

Scaife, J. (2019). *Supervision in clinical practice: a practitioner's guide* (3rd ed.). Milton Park, Abingdon, Oxon: Routledge.

Searles, H. F. (1955). The informational value of the supervisor's emotional experiences. *Psychiatry, 18*(2), 135–146.

Simpson-Southward, C., Waller, G., & Hardy, G. E. (2017). How do we know what makes for "best practice" in clinical supervision for psychological therapists? A content analysis of supervisory models and approaches. *Clinical Psychology & Psychotherapy, 24*(6), 1228–1245.

Stoltenberg, C. (1981). Approaching supervision from a developmental perspective: The counselor complexity model. *Journal of Counseling Psychology, 28*(1), 59.

Stoltenberg, C., & McNeill, B. (2011). *IDM supervision: An integrative developmental model for supervising counselors and therapists.* New York: Routledge.

Stoltenberg, C., McNeill, B., & Delworth, U. (1988). *IDM: An integrated developmental model for supervising counselors and therapists.* San Francisco: Josey-Bass.

Stoltenberg, C., Bailey, K. C., Cruzan, C. B., Hart, J. T., & Ukuku, U. (2014). The integrative developmental model of supervision. In C. E. Watkins Jr & D. Milne (Eds.), *The Wiley international handbook of clinical supervision* (pp. 576–597). Malden, MA: Wiley.

Chapter 4

The "Educating function"

Learning the EMDR protocol

- Kolb's "Learning Cycle"
- Learning styles
- The "LEAP" Model
- Reflective practice
- Building on the supervisee's existing knowledge
- Learning from mistakes
- Teaching by telling stories and self-disclosure
- From training to supervision
- Mistakes made by EMDR supervisees
- Competence
- Metacompetence
- Not just teaching the protocol
- Do we need to know every protocol?
- Backing up session with resources

This chapter and the following two chapters will be organised according to each of the three basic functions of clinical supervision as described in Chapter 3:

- Educating
- Enabling
- Evaluating

We start in this chapter with the "formative" function (Proctor, 1988), which I prefer to describe as the "Educating" function of supervision. In terms of EMDR, this is very much about learning the EMDR Standard Protocol and developing the necessary skills to utilise EMDR with one's clients. Whilst the supervisor plays a crucial role in this, the learning process obviously starts on the first morning of the supervisee's basic EMDR training. The following account will therefore attempt to integrate what happens in training with what occurs during supervision.

To begin with, let us go back to basics and look at the nature of educating and learning generally before we apply this specifically to EMDR

DOI: 10.4324/9781003214588-5

supervision. Bear in mind, however, that the AIP model is, in itself, a theory about learning. I will therefore attempt to incorporate insights relating to the AIP model as I review the literature on the nature of teaching and learning.

Kolb's "learning cycle"

Let me start by relating my own experience of reading Kolb's seminal work, *Experiential Learning* (Kolb, 2015). As I started to work my way through this book, I first tried to make sense of what Kolb was saying, putting it into my own words and understanding it in relation to what I already think is happening when people are trained and supervised in EMDR therapy. I started to think about what is taking place, for example, when an experienced CBT therapist first observes a session of EMDR therapy during their Part 1 training and how they try to assimilate this with what they already understand about therapy. For example, they might be wondering how cognitive change could be occurring in the absence of Socratic Questioning.

Kolb talks of learning as an interaction between the person and their environment and regards learning as the major process of human adaptation. He makes no mention of Attachment Theory but clearly the type of attachment style that an infant develops at an early age reflects their best attempts at adapting to the world in which they find themselves in order to maximise their safety (Bowlby, 1969).

Kolb refers to the work of Piaget (1970) who posited that the key to learning lay in the mutual interaction of the process of "accommodation" of concepts or schemas to experiences in the world and the process of "assimilation" of events and experiences from the world into existing concepts and schemas. Kolb describes the experiential "learning cycle," where he defines learning as "the process whereby knowledge is created through the transformation of experience" (Kolb, 2015, p. 51). He describes knowledge as resulting from the combination of taking in information and then transforming the experience. The latter is the way in which individuals interpret and act on the information they have taken in. He describes four learning modes as follows:

- Concrete experience
- Reflective observation
- Abstract conceptualisation
- Active experimentation

Immediate or concrete experiences are the basis for observations and reflections. These reflections are assimilated and distilled into abstract concepts from which new implications for action can be drawn. These implications can be actively tested and serve as guides in creating new experiences.

(Kolb, 2015, p. 51)

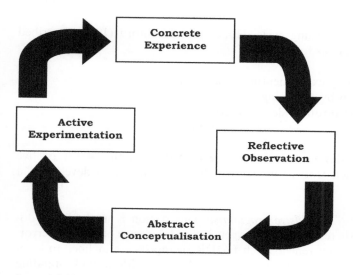

Figure 4.1 Kolb's leaning cycle (Kolb, 2015).

Figure 4.1 summarises Kolb's "learning cycle."

Compare this to the AIP model which describes the way in which we process new experiences and assimilate them into our existing understanding of ourselves and the world. When we are able to adaptively process an experience in this way, "we learn something about ourselves and other people, we better understand past situations, and we are better able to handle similar situations in the future" (Shapiro, 2018, p. 27). Kolb's model appears to be compatible with the AIP model and provides more detail about the process by which this learning and adaptation happen. This is particularly relevant in understanding what occurs when someone is training in a new therapy such as EMDR.

Let us think about what is happening as the trainee sits on the first day of basic EMDR training and is being told about the AIP model and how this relates to the EMDR Standard Protocol. It starts with *concrete experience* of what the trainer is presenting. The trainee will then reflect (*reflective observation*) on what they have been told and start to assimilate this with what they already understand about psychological functioning and their own experience as a therapist. They will then move on to creating some new abstract concepts (*abstract conceptualisation*) as a result of this assimilation helped, perhaps, by questions they may ask of the trainer. Finally, they will experience using EMDR therapy themselves in the training (*active experimentation*) either as a client or as a therapist which, itself, is a further concrete experience. And so the cycle goes on.

Learning styles

Building on Kolb's learning cycle, Honey and Mumford (1992) described four "learning styles" as follows:

• Activists – learn by experimenting with new ideas
• Reflectors – learn by observing and thinking
• Theorists – learn through ideas and concepts
• Pragmatists – learn by applying ideas to practice

Hawkins and McMahon (2020) have developed from this a list of five learning styles which tend to limit the individuals' ability to develop as a therapist:

• *The fire-fighter – compulsive pragmatist*: This person is in the "plan-do-plan-do" trap where learning never gets beyond the stage of trial and error. This person does not reflect. Such EMDR therapists are inclined to learn and try a host of different protocols and techniques without understanding the importance of case conceptualisation.
• *The post-mortemiser*: The "reflect-do-reflect-do" trap. This person is restricting their approach to correcting errors without actually learning from them and generalising to their development as a therapist.
• *The navel-gazing theorist*: The "reflect-theorise-reflect-theorise" trap. These therapists are adept at understanding their client in great depth and may be excellent at case conceptualisation. However, they tend not to actually "crack on" and may be reluctant to commence Phase 4 processing in EMDR.
• *The paralysis by analysis*: The trap is "analyse-plan-then-analyse-some-more." Learning is limited by fear and, similar to the navel-gazing theorist, this EMDR therapist may never get started with processing.
• *The totalitarian*: The "theorise-do" trap, where the motto is "work it out in private and then impose it on them." This means the therapist is unlikely to be flexible enough to respond to what is happening in the session.

When one thinks specifically about how this applies to EMDR supervision, there are some important considerations. If the supervisee is a pragmatist, they are likely to have little difficulty in getting stuck into doing EMDR processing. However, they may need more help with case conceptualisation, standing back and reflecting on what is happening with their client. If they are a theorist, they will need more help with being able to act and experience and get going with Phase 4 processing.

Fear is often the reason why particular therapists become stuck in a particular learning style. Over many years the individual will have developed their learning style as their own "safe place" when they feel under pressure.

Kolb (2015) describes these as "nonlearning postures." Learning a new therapy such as EMDR may drive them back into their safe place. Pepper (1942) shows that the extreme positions of "dogmatism" and "absolute scepticism" are inadequate foundations for learning. He proposes that "partial scepticism" is more conducive to learning.

The "LEAP" model

Of particular relevance to EMDR is the Longitudinal Education for Advancing Practice (LEAP) model (McLeod et al., 2018) which was developed in order to look specifically at the training of individuals in an evidence-based therapy (EBT). They point out that, in isolation, training strategies produce small effects and therefore need to be followed up by ongoing "consultation."

Drawing on the work of Bennett-Levy (2006) and others, the model looks at three "cognitive-based mechanisms" involved in learning as follows:

- Declarative
- Procedural
- Reflective

Declarative

The first step in the learning process is acquiring *declarative knowledge* (i.e. factual knowledge and information about a therapy). Changes in declarative knowledge are expected to occur as a result of an initial training, or soon thereafter. Put into simple language, this is the stage of learning facts about the new therapy.

The transfer of learning process begins as trainees form *procedural knowledge* (i.e. knowledge about how to deliver a therapy) and decision-making *heuristics* that are used to organise and guide the application of the emerging knowledge. This will develop as trainees start their EMDR practice, allowing them to determine how skills and knowledge can be used together to achieve goals.

Procedural

Two cognitive processes, *proceduralisation* and *composition* (Anderson, 1982) are instrumental to the formation of heuristics. In *proceduralisation*, a trainee identifies and organises the discrete steps required to deliver a therapy into a larger routine, for example, using a worksheet in order to be guided through the Assessment Phase of the EMDR protocol. In *composition*, a trainee groups the steps by linking them into a more complex process. Applying procedural knowledge and developing heuristics requires cognitive resources.

Trainees often describe their use of EMDR as being "clunky" at this stage as they need to think through each small step in using EMDR and are pre-occupied with the protocol.

Reflective

As trainees gain experience, they develop faster, more sophisticated heuristics for organising information. They internalise the application of knowledge and form habits. Once internalised, fewer cognitive resources are required to perform a task, leaving the individual free to apply their attention elsewhere such as tracking client emotion during processing. Metacognition – the awareness and regulation of one's own cognitive processes and the effects of one's behaviour on others – is developed during this phase (Brown, 1975; Leonesio & Nelson, 1990). This allows trainees to track progress towards accomplishing goals, determine when an approach is not working, and problem-solve while delivering interventions during a treatment session. Bennett-Levy (2006) called this the "reflective" system and suggested that it plays a key role in helping clinicians determine how and when to use specific clinical interventions. Cognitive strategies play a role in helping clinicians generalise knowledge to new situations, which is central to becoming a competent clinician.

Reflective practice

Developing the theme of the third cognitive-based mechanism above, I will now look in more detail at reflective practice. Schon (1983) defines reflective practice as "the capacity to reflect on action so as to engage in a process of continuous learning" (p. 68). He distinguishes two types of reflection:

- Reflection-on-action
- Reflection-in-action

Reflection-on-action occurs after a therapy session when the therapist reviews their work either alone or in discussion with a colleague such as their supervisor. However, therapists need to also make moment-by-moment decisions during a therapy session which Shon refers to as *reflection-in-action*.

Reflective practice also includes "self-knowledge, which includes the capacity to think about what you bring to the work, your own values, beliefs, thoughts, and feelings" (Beinart & Clohessy, 2017, p. 125). These authors also refer to Dewey (1933) who said that reflective open-mindedness includes the ability to "recognize the possibility of error even in the beliefs that are dearest to us" (p. 29).

Research suggests that poor supervisors spend too much time on case-focused discussions and insufficient time on supervisee-focused outcomes or on the process of learning (Inman & Ladany, 2008). "We need to create a learning climate ... that supports our supervisees in taking a step back to make sense of their own experiences rather than going through endless descriptive retellings of their work" (Beinart & Clohessy, 2017, p. 126). This is reflected in the mantra from EMDR Consultants' Trainings to "teach from the theory."

Building on the supervisee's existing knowledge

I have already referred to the fact that all our supervisees will have trained and, in many cases, be very experienced in some other therapeutic modality. As supervisors teaching the EMDR protocol, it is important that we always acknowledge where our supervisees are coming from and to start from there. For example, when teaching about therapeutic interweaves I have had comments from CBT therapists that it sounds rather like CBT to which I will reply, "an interweave *is* like a little bit of CBT that we are throwing in here, but the difference is that we then stay out of the way and trust the process and only use another interweave if they get stuck again."

"There is a good deal of evidence that learning is enhanced when teachers pay attention to the knowledge and beliefs that learners bring to a learning task, use this knowledge as a starting point for new instruction, and monitor students' changing conceptions as instruction proceeds" (Bransford, Brown, & Cocking, 2000, p. 11).

Learning from mistakes

One day I was puzzling over one note in a saxophone run that Branford had played and I thought, "one of these notes is wrong. Which one is it?" And Gill [Evans] turned to me and said "Sting, there's no such thing as a wrong note." I said, "what do you mean Gill?" He said, "It's the note that follows what you think of as a mistake because that is the note that can open up a whole world of opportunity and a world of potential that you hadn't realised before. It's how you react to a mistake." And of course, you take that as a philosophy of life. All of us make mistakes, you know, wrong decisions here and there. It's how you react to that event which marks whether it's successful or not.

(Sting, 2021)

Therapists are often scared of making mistakes, perhaps particularly in EMDR when many suspect that they are secretly getting it all wrong. So, this is an important issue to address.

"Success is a lousy teacher," said Bill Gates. In my trainings and supervision, I always emphasise that, when we make a mistake, we learn more than when we get things right the first time. I also quote the conductor of my choir who says that, when you get to a tricky bit that you are unsure about, "sing up so I can hear your mistakes and help to correct you." We never "fail" as therapists. We just learn more about our client and the therapy we are using. If something goes wrong, it is new information, not a disaster. In fact, there is some experimental evidence to indicate that actually making deliberate errors in a learning task will enhance the learning (Wong & Lim, 2022).

It is also important to model openness about errors in therapy by disclosing one's own and, in my own case, I have plenty to choose from! Experimental studies have shown that the greater the perceived similarity, the greater the imitation. A famous study by Meichenbaum (1971) used film models who were initially anxious but overcame their anxiety ("coping model"), resulting in greater anxiety reduction in viewers than those whose models were completely fearless ("mastery model"). "Supervisors may disclose the many errors they have made in the course of their career. This type of disclosure creates the norm of admitting mistakes, models coping, and facilitates identification" (Friedberg et al., 2009, p. 115). Claxton (1987) describes the four beliefs that get in the way of adult learning:

- I must be competent
- I must be in control
- I must be consistent
- I must be comfortable

Hawkins and McMahon (2020) say that we must set a climate that challenges these beliefs. To do so, we must avoid appearing as "super-competent in-control experts," but rather as experienced supervisors who are still open to learning and are open about our vulnerabilities.

Be aware, however, that there may be cultural issues here. For example, amongst some Asian therapists there would be an expectation that the supervisor should be infallible and that it would be a weakness to admit to any mistakes.

Teaching by telling stories and self-disclosure

I have been surprised by the apparent absence in the literature about the use of one's own stories of therapy as a device for teaching supervisees. Whilst some writers have discussed the way in which cases in supervision are presented through storytelling (Carroll, 2014) or how classic fairy stories can be used to illustrate the dilemmas that our clients face (Ward & Sommer, 2006), writers on supervision do not refer to how supervisors tell their supervisees stories about their own practice.

Rather than respond with direct advice to my supervisees about how they might proceed with a particular client who they are presenting in supervision, I will tend to tell a story about a similar client who I have worked with. Often the story will include a description of the mistakes that I have made in order to model that it is OK to get things wrong and to be open about this (see previous section). The story also helps the supervisee to generalise from their own particular case and to develop their own response as to how to proceed with their client based on the message contained within the story. I have occasionally checked with my supervisees as to whether they find my storytelling useful. I have always had a positive response and one supervisee said, "I love hearing your stories, Robin, particularly the ones about when you have messed up!"

Whilst I have not discovered any specific research evidence regarding the effectiveness of this in the supervision literature, there is some evidence in relation to education in general. In classrooms, a teacher's use of narratives, humour, and self-disclosure has been found to be an effective tool in helping students to understand the material (Downs, Javidi, & Nussbaum, 1988). In an experimental study by Kromka and Goodboy (2019), the lesson given to the experimental group concluded with a story which summarised the content of the lesson. As compared to the control group, students in the narrative lecture condition liked the instructor more, reported more sustained attention toward the lecture, performed slightly better on a test of short-term recall and performed better on a retention test of extraneous information. Instructors who disclose relevant and appropriate personal information increase perceptions of caring, instructor credibility, and affinity with students' experiences (Myers, Brann, & Members of Comm 600, 2009).

From training to supervision

One of the unique aspects of EMDR supervision is the way in which it is closely linked to the basic training. I have already referred to this in Chapter 1. At a very illuminating day-long workshop by Bruce Perry at the EMDR Europe conference in The Hague in 2016 (Perry, 2016) I learned an important lesson about the nature of how we learn: However, excellent your teaching is, students will not absorb all the information because, whilst they are processing and assimilating one piece of information, they will not have the capacity to take in what you tell them next. This accords with the AIP model and the idea that we do not just make a video recording of our experience, but we assimilate it with our existing experience and knowledge. In a training situation, where a trainee is learning about EMDR for the first time, they will need to make sense of what they are learning by assimilating it with how they already understand psychological functioning and therapy. Therefore, even a supervisee who is intelligent, attentive and diligent and has trained with the best trainer will still have gaps in their knowledge which the supervisor will need to find as they go along.

I have already referred to the essential differences between training and supervision in Chapter 1 and need to return to this here. Table 4.1 is based on Milne (2018).

Table 4.1 The differences between training and supervision

	Training	Supervision
Agenda	Determined by the trainer	Supervisee dictates it
Objective	To learn basics of EMDR therapy	To develop expertise in using EMDR
Values	Conformity and compliance	Challenge and change

Source: Based on Milne (2018).

Essentially training is led by the trainer whilst supervision is led by the learner. Having said this, there are some ways in which the supervisor does lead supervision. They provide the structure for the supervisee to learn, rather like the therapist provides structure for the client.

As described above in the section on the LEAP model, during the basic training, trainees will be at the stages of *declarative knowledge* and moving into *procedural knowledge*. As supervisors we will be picking them up, expecting them to be already mastering *procedural knowledge* and moving into the *reflective* stage. But with many supervisees, particularly at an early stage, we will still be "mopping up" on the *declarative* stage and finding gaps in their understanding of the Standard Protocol. These gaps may still be apparent when they attend the Consultants' Training, the first day of which involves brushing up on the Standard Protocol. Even facilitators (and on the rare occasion, dare I say it, myself as a trainer!) discover finer points of the Standard Protocol that we may have misunderstood.

Mistakes made by EMDR supervisees

Derek Farrell, at an online workshop regarding EMDR supervision (Farrell, 2020), described the five "Most common occurring 'mistakes' identified in EMDR Therapy Clinical Supervision" as follows:

- Insufficient History Taking
- Deficient AIP case conceptualisation
- Lack of a robust Target Treatment Plan
- Not enough Preparation: Stabilisation and Resource Installation
- Too much Preparation

The first two of these, relate to *"History Taking"* and *"AIP case conceptualisation"* (Ploszajski, 2021). Some supervisees can get bogged down with the technicalities of the EMDR protocol which prevents them from standing back and looking at the big picture. As one of my supervisees described it, sometimes "you need to keep your oar out of the water." When formulation is correct, the course of action becomes obvious. In my experience, this sometimes relates to the professional background of the EMDR therapist. For example, a clinical psychologist will have a background in comprehensive History Taking and case conceptualisation. In contrast, someone with a background in counselling will have received less training in this area. Supervisors will often need to assist supervisees to develop their skills in this area. A useful framework in relation to case conceptualisation is Ines Santos's "Case Formulation Tool" (Santos, 2019). This uses visual representation, based on a series of boxes which can be filled in, to capture and simplify the AIP approach to case formulation. Visual representation is useful to capture different elements and how they relate to each other and also to share formulation with the client. The six key elements of Santos's AIP Case Formulation Tool are as follows:

- Trauma(s) (unprocessed traumatic memories)
- Triggers
- Intrusions (intrusive memories, flashbacks/nightmares, sensory memories including pain)
- Negative beliefs (four domains)
- Symptoms/behaviours/difficulties
- Resilience factors (positive experiences, positive attachment figures [past and present], strengths, achievements, current positives in life [strong marriage, parenting, career, hobbies])

AIP case formulation is a process of establishing relationships between these six elements and drawing causative arrows between elements, showing how unprocessed events cause current symptoms.

The third of Farrell's "common mistakes" is *"lack of a robust Target Treatment Plan."* Frequently in supervision, the mistake relates not to an adequate history taking and case formulation but a difficulty in finding the "hot" target for processing. One of the issues here is that supervisees often go for the obvious target rather than the target that taps into the client's current pathology. In my trainings, there is a story that I tell, which will illustrate this. It is about a client who was sexually abused by a neighbour as a child. However, it was not the sexual abuse itself which we targeted in EMDR therapy. Her mother's hostile reaction and denial that it could have taken place when it was disclosed to her was what had most affected my client. Our target memory was therefore her mother's reaction to the disclosure rather than the sexual abuse itself. Often the best way of teaching this is to tell a story about one's own practice which illustrates this point.

Next comes *"Not enough Preparation: Stabilisation and Resource Installation."* Some supervisees make the mistake of rushing in too early without ensuring that their client is ready to start processing. I have to confess that this is something I have been guilty of in my time. Here it is useful to go back to some basic teaching about the Standard Protocol and the importance of the Preparation Phase. As a framework for this in my own teaching, I utilise Joany Spierings's "Milkstool Test" (Spierings, 2008). This describes the three kinds of basic resources that are required to tolerate EMDR processing. These would normally be developed at an early age through interaction with one's attachment figure as part of developing a secure attachment. They can be seen as the three legs of a milking stool: without any one of its three legs, the stool would collapse. The three "legs" are as follows:

• Affect regulation: An ability to regulate one's emotions
• Inner connectedness: A sense that there is someone else out there to whom you matter, a "go to person"
• Self-image: Experiencing yourself as someone who has the right to exist

Through preparation and resource installation, I impress upon my supervisees the importance of all three "legs" being in place before they start processing any traumatic memories.

Finally, on the list of Farrell's common mistakes is *"Too much Preparation."* This will usually occur as a result of the supervisee's lack of confidence in relation to using EMDR. Here, the issue is not one of the Educating function (teaching the EMDR protocol) which is the subject of this chapter. It comes instead under the "Enabling" function which is the subject of the next chapter.

Competence

"Competence" appears to be a 21st-century buzzword in relation to the training of psychological therapies. EMDR Europe specifies a "competency-based framework" as being the gold standard against which we measure our supervisees' suitability for accreditation. (This will be discussed in more detail in relation to the accreditation process in Chapter 6.) Meanwhile the NHS in England has developed competency frameworks for a number of therapies including EMDR (Roth, Dudley, & Pilling, 2021). So, what do we mean by "competence"?

> Competence refers to an individual's capability and demonstrated ability to understand and do certain tasks in an appropriate and effective manner consistent with the expectations for a person qualified by education and training in a particular profession or specialty thereof.
>
> (Kaslow et al., 2004, p. 775)

However, the state of competence "is not an absolute, nor does it involve a narrow set of professional behaviors; rather competence reflects sufficiency of a broad spectrum of personal and professional abilities relative to a given requirement" (Falender & Shafranske, 2004, p. 5). In addition to the actual performance of a specific clinical skill, "competence" indicates the motivation and action to achieve a level of capability and is therefore essential to continuous professional development, which ensures competence (Falender & Shafranske, 2007).

Paradoxically, some authors have suggested that the competency-based approach does not actually reflect competence and "fails to take account of the real character of professionalism on the one hand and the artistry of practice on the other" (Fish & de Cossart, 2006, p. 404). Corrie and Lane (2015) warn us against becoming too bogged down with competency frameworks and quote Gambrill (2007) who cautions that, if competencies are divorced from the decision-making process, there is a risk of "bucket theory"-thinking, where the task of training becomes conceptualised as one of pouring knowledge into the trainees' heads.

Metacompetence

"Give a man a fish, and you feed him for a day. Teach a man to fish, and you feed him for a lifetime."

(Anon)

One of the mantras on the EMDR trainings is about "teaching from the theory." Rather than tell our supervisees what to do with a particular client, we take them back to the AIP model and explain the theoretical basis for what we are saying to our supervisees.

Metacompetence, or "knowing what one knows and what one does not know" (Falender & Shafranske, 2007, p. 235), refers to the use of available skills and knowledge to solve problems or tasks and to determine which skills or knowledge are missing, how to acquire these, and whether they are essential to success. A prerequisite to metacompetence is the ability to introspect about one's personal cognitive processes and products and is dependent on self-awareness, self-reflection, and self-assessment (Weinert, 2001). Supervision clearly plays an essential role in guiding the development of metacompetence.

Bernard's "Discrimination Model" (Bernard, 1979, 1997) may be useful to develop the idea of metacompetence and how it can be engendered in our supervisees. The model describes three possible foci for supervision as well as three possible roles for the supervisor. The three foci are as follows:

- Intervention: What the supervisee is doing in the therapy session?
- Conceptualisation: How the supervisee understands what is occurring?
- Personalisation: How the supervisee's own personal style interfaces with their way of working with clients?

To my mind these foci overlap, to a certain extent, with some of the "eyes" in the Seven-Eyed model (Hawkins, 1985). The second of these, "conceptualisation" is important because, as we stress at the EMDR Consultants training, we need to "teach from the theory" so that supervisees can generalise what they have learned, rather than just being told what to do with a particular client.

The three roles that can be adopted by the supervisor are as follows:

- Teacher: Instruction, modelling and direct feedback
- Counsellor: Helping the supervisee to be reflective, focussing on their internal affect
- Consultant: More collegial, encouraging the supervisee to trust their own insights and feelings about their work, or challenging supervisees to think and act on their own

One can see that as the supervisor moves into the second and third of these roles, the supervisee is starting to learn to become metacompetent and move beyond just learning the Standard Protocol of EMDR.

As Gordon (2012) points out, we are aiming to follow Kolb's cycle of adult learning (Kolb, 2015) by moving from concrete experience to observation and reflection. A further question such as, "What can you learn from this to help with future clients?" will help move the supervisee on to Kolb's next stage, namely the formation of more abstract conceptualisations and generalisations.

My own experience of how this will actually feel during a session of supervision is that there will be a noticeable cognitive and emotional shift in the supervisee when they have learned something new. Their apparent discomfort with their, as yet, unresolved Supervision Question will give way to an expression of relief as if to say "aha!" and, if we are lucky, an expression of gratitude!

Not just teaching the protocol

As EMDR supervisors we must remember that, even in terms of the "Educating" function of supervision, our job is often not just to teach the Standard Protocol of EMDR. Although there is a requirement that, prior to training in EMDR, all trainees are fully trained and experienced psychological therapists, it often becomes apparent during supervision that some supervisees lack some of the basic skills that we would expect them to have.

Sometimes this is in relation to case formulation which I have already discussed. Sometimes it will be shortcomings in developing a therapeutic relationship with the client which is a prerequisite to the effectiveness of EMDR when we start processing. The supervisee may need some specific instruction and feedback about their posture, facial expression, tone of voice or receptiveness to changes in emotion in the client. They need to ensure that the client can feel safe and in control during the therapy session and that, during the Desensitisation Phase, their principal role is to "bear witness."

Do we need to know every protocol?

An EMDR Consultant, who I supervise, was worried because she felt that she needed to have all the protocols for EMDR at her fingertips in order to answer her supervisees' questions. Well, that would be an impossibility. Firstly, we should never let go of the fact that the Standard Protocol can be applied to any situation. There is a tendency for some EMDR therapists to think that they need a specific protocol for every psychological disorder and that, if they are not working with PTSD, they need to use some different protocol. When expressing her irritation with this tendency at the UK annual EMDR conference in 2019, Anabel Gonzalez said, "all we need is the Standard Protocol and some common sense!" I would fully concur with this although we do have specific protocols, for example for pain or recent events, which have quite distinct characteristics and which our supervisees may need to learn.

As an EMDR supervisor, I cannot be fully conversant with every protocol that exists. But I should have an overview of the available protocols and keep a virtual library of papers and handouts in relation to these protocols (see next section). I have been told that one well-known supervisor simply says, "I can't help you because that's not my area of expertise." I believe that is not good enough and that, as a supervisor, I need to say instead, "I don't know the answer, but I think I know where to find it. I will get back to you on this one."

Backing up session with resources

Although one of our functions as supervisors is to teach, we do not necessarily need to do all of this within the confines of a supervision session. If, for example, I have explained a specific protocol to a supervisee I will follow up the session with an academic paper, handout, PowerPoint presentation, or weblink attached to an email in order that they can do some further reading on the topic and have a written protocol to follow. This is generally much appreciated by my supervisees. It is therefore important as a supervisor to start building up a library of resources to share with supervisees.

Conclusion

This chapter has focused on the "Educating" function of supervision and started by looking at theories about adult learning and how these relate to the AIP model which is, itself, a learning model. By being aware of *how* they learn, we can, as supervisors, enhance the way in which our supervisees learn about the EMDR protocol and use EMDR in their therapeutic work.

Anderson, J. R. (1982). Acquisition of cognitive skill. *Psychological Review*, *89*(4), 369.

Beinart, H., & Clohessy, S. (2017). *Effective supervisory relationships. Best evidence and practice*. Chichester, UK: Wiley.

Bennett-Levy, J. (2006). Therapist skills: A cognitive model of their acquisition and refinement. *Behavioural and Cognitive Psychotherapy*, *34*(1), 57–78.

Bernard, J. M. (1979). Supervisor training: A discrimination model. *Counselor Education and Supervision*, *19*(1), 60–68.

Bernard, J. M. (1997). The discrimination model. In C. Watkins (Ed.), *Handbook of psychotherapy supervision* (pp. 310–327). New York: NY: Wiley.

Bowlby, J. (1969). *Attachment and loss, volume 1: Attachment*. London: Hogarth Press and The Institute of Psycho-Analysis.

Bransford, J. D., Brown, A. L., & Cocking, R. R. (2000). *How people learn: Brain, mind, experience, and school*. Washington, DC: National Academy Press.

Brown, A. L. (1975). The development of memory: Knowing, knowing about knowing, and knowing how to know. *Advances in Child Development and Behavior*, *10*, 103–152.

Carroll, M. (2014). *Effective supervision for the helping professions* (2nd ed.). London: Sage.

Claxton, G. (1987). *Live and learn: An introduction to the psychology of growth and change in everyday life*. Maidenhead: Open University Press.

Corrie, S., & Lane, D. (2015). *CBT supervision*. London: Sage.

Dewey, J. (1933). *How we think*. Buffalo, NY: Promethius.

Downs, V., Javidi, M., & Nussbaum, J. (1988). An analysis of teachers' verbal communication within the college classroom: Use of humor, self-disclosure, and narratives. *Communication Education*, *37*(2), 127–141.

Falender, C. A., & Shafranske, E. P. (2004). Clinical supervision: A competency-based approach. PDF retrieved from www.cfalender.com

Falender, C. A., & Shafranske, E. P. (2007). Competence in competency-based supervision practice: Construct and application. *Professional Psychology: Research and Practice*, *38*(3), 232.

Farrell, D. (2020). *Advanced clinical supervision and consultation skills in enhancing competency in EMDR therapy*. EMDR Lebanon Association.

Fish, D., & de Cossart, L. (2006). Thinking outside the (tick) box: Rescuing professionalism and professional judgement. *Medical Education*, *40*(5), 404–406.

Friedberg, R. D., Gorman, A. A., & Beidel, D. C. (2009). Training psychologists for cognitive-behavioral therapy in the raw world: A rubric for supervisors. *Behavior Modification*, *33*(1), 104–123.

Gambrill, E. (2007). Transparency as the route to evidence-informed professional education. *Research on Social Work Practice*, *17*(5), 553–560.

Gordon, P. (2012). Ten steps to cognitive behavioural supervision. *The Cognitive Behaviour Therapist*, *5*(4), 71–82.

Hawkins, P. (1985). Humanistic psychotherapy supervision: A conceptual framework. *Self & Society*, *13*(2), 69–76.

Hawkins, P., & McMahon, A. (2020). *Supervision in the helping professions* (5th ed.). London: Open University Press.

Honey, P., & Mumford, A. (1992). *The manual of learning styles (Vol. 3)*. Maidenhead, UK: Peter Honey.

Inman, A., & Ladany, N. (2008). Research: The state of the field. *Psychotherapy Supervison: Theory Research and Practice, 2*, 500–517.

Kaslow, N. J., Borden, K. A., Collins Jr, F. L., Forrest, L., Illfelder-Kaye, J., Nelson, P. D., ... Willmuth, M. E. (2004). Competencies conference: Future directions in education and credentialing in professional psychology. *Journal of Clinical Psychology, 60*(7), 699–712.

Kolb, D. (2015). *Experiential learning: Experience as the source of learning and development* (2nd ed.). New Jersey: Pearson.

Kromka, S. M., & Goodboy, A. K. (2019). Classroom storytelling: Using instructor narratives to increase student recall, affect, and attention. *Communication Education, 68*(1), 20–43.

Leonesio, R. J., & Nelson, T. O. (1990). Do different metamemory judgments tap the same underlying aspects of memory? *Journal of Experimental Psychology: Learning, Memory, and Cognition, 16*(3), 464.

McLeod, B. D., Cox, J. R., Jensen-Doss, A., Herschell, A., Ehrenreich-May, J., & Wood, J. J. (2018). Proposing a mechanistic model of clinician training and consultation. *Clinical Psychology: Science and Practice, 25*(3), e12260.

Meichenbaum, D. H. (1971). Examination of model characteristics in reducing avoidance behavior. *Journal of Personality and Social Psychology, 17*(3), 298.

Milne, D. (2018). *Evidence-based CBT supervision: principles and practice* (2nd ed.). Hoboken, NJ: Wiley.

Myers, S., Brann, M., & Members of Comm 600. (2009). College students' perceptions of how instructors establish and enhance credibility through self-disclosure. *Qualitative Research Reports in Communication, 10*(1), 9–16.

Pepper, S. C. (1942). *World hypotheses: A study in evidence* (Vol. 31): London: Univ. California Press.

Perry, B. (2016). *Introduction to the neurosequential model of therapeutics*. Paper presented at the 17th European EMDR conference, The Hague.

Piaget, J. (1970). *The place of the sciences of man in the system of science*. New York: Harper Torchbooks.

Ploszajski, J. (2021). Seeing the wood and the trees: a pilot study of the clinical value and ease of use of four approaches to case formulation. *EMDR Therapy Quarterly, 3*(4).

Proctor, B. (1988). Supervision: a co-operative exercise in accountability. In M. Marken, & M. Payne (Eds.), *Enabling and ensuring*. Leicester: National Youth Bureau and Council for Education and Training in Youth and Community Work.

Roth, A., Dudley, O., & Pilling, S. (2021). *A competence framework for eye movement desensitisation and reprocessing (EMDR) therapy*. London: University College London.

Santos, I. (2019). EMDR case formulation tool. *Journal of EMDR Practice and Research, 13*(3), 221–231.

Schon, D. (1983). *The reflective practitioner*. New York: Basic Books.

Shapiro, F. (2018). *Eye movement desensitization and reprocessing (EMDR) Therapy: Basic principles, protocols, and procedures* (3rd ed.). New York: Guilford Publications.

Spierings, J. (2008). Stabilisatie, een gestructureerd programma voor taxatie en interventie. In E. ten Broeke, A. de Jongh, & H. Oppenheim (Eds.), *Praktijkboek EMDR*. Amsterdam: Pearson Assessment and Information.

Sting. (2021). This cultural life. *BBC Radio 4*.

Ward, J. E., & Sommer, C. A. (2006). Using stories in supervision to facilitate counselor development. *Journal of Poetry Therapy, 19*(2), 61–67.

Weinert, F. E. (2001). Concept of competence: A conceptual clarification. In D. S. Rychen & L. H. Salganik (Eds.), *Defining and selecting key competencies*. Seattle, WA: Hogrefe & Huber.

Wong, S. S. H., & Lim, S. W. H. (2022). The derring effect: Deliberate errors enhance learning. *Journal of Experimental Psychology: General, 151*(1), 25.

The "Enabling" function
Enabling and supporting the therapist

- The supervisory relationship
- Trust and supervisor self-disclosure
- Supervisee self-disclosure
- The parallel process
- Telling my story
- The power relationship
- Trainees will not practise EMDR without supervision

My first meeting with a new supervisee

Initially, she seemed to be rather guarded with me, not surprising, given that this was our first meeting. During the introductory preamble, I was asking her about her professional background and experience. I also asked her about her theoretical orientation. When she started to tell me about this, it reminded me of my own history and why EMDR seemed to be what I was looking for when I first encountered it. I therefore briefly shared my own story with her. Sharing of my own experience appeared to punctuate the meeting and produce a marked change. She started speaking much more openly and warmly about how she works and how EMDR might fit into her theoretical orientation. She appeared to be more at ease with me and it suddenly felt as if we had skipped several sessions and now knew each other well.

I wondered afterwards how my spontaneous sharing of my own experience had impacted our supervisory relationship. My guess is that it served two functions: Firstly, it took the pressure off my supervisee and, for the first time in the meeting, the focus was not on her. Secondly, I was modelling for her that it is OK to share one's own doubts and realisations in relation to the therapeutic work that we do.

The great range of activities that make up the daily interaction between a mother and her baby can be seen to fall roughly into four dimensions:

DOI: 10.4324/9781003214588-6

- Structure
- Engagement
- Nurture
- Challenge

(Booth & Jernberg, 2010, p. 20)

The above quote comes from a textbook on Theraplay, an attachment-based therapy for children. It strikes me that these four basic dimensions are also those that are crucial for a successful and effective supervisory relationship.

We now move on to looking at the second of the three basic functions of supervision, namely Proctor's (1988) "restorative" function – or the "Enabling" function as I prefer to call it. The Enabling function is about supporting our supervisees with the emotional effects of their work, in particular with those clients in acute distress. But it is also about helping our supervisees with their own uncertainty and lack of confidence regarding their practice as EMDR therapists. My experience as a trainer is that some trainees never start EMDR therapy with their clients because they have been unable to access supervision. For them, at the start of their EMDR career, the Enabling function of supervision is probably what they have lacked more than anything else.

"It is important to be aware that the supervisory room is crowded with all sorts of 'persons' who create anxieties for both the supervisor and the supervisee" (Lesser, 1983, p. 126). Underlying this is always a fear of being judged; this holds true both for supervisee and supervisor. Even after practising EMDR myself for more than two decades, having been president of the EMDR Association UK, an EMDR trainer and a teacher on Consultant's Trainings, when I am receiving supervision myself, I always approach it with some trepidation. A little fear is a good thing and, I believe, signals an acceptance that one might be challenged by one's supervisor.

The supervisory relationship

The most important starting place for this chapter, in my view, is to look at the supervisory relationship.

In their analysis of what makes a "competent clinical supervisor," Roth and Pilling (2008) found that the "supervisory alliance" emerged as a basic building block of successful supervision. In a meta-analysis of 40 studies, Watkins (2014) concluded that the "supervisory alliance" is consistently the crucial component of a successful supervisory relationship. Compare this with the well-established research evidence to show that the therapeutic relationship has more impact on outcome than the actual therapy utilised (Baier, Kline, & Feeny, 2020).

Let us begin with a seminal paper by Edward Bordin regarding the "Working Alliance Based Model of Supervision" (Bordin, 1983). Drawing on the concept of the "working alliance" in therapy, he describes three main aspects:

- *Mutual agreements:* regarding the goals of supervision
- *Tasks*: how the supervision will be done
- *Bonds:* the emotional connection (including trust).

Bordin suggests that time spent together, mutual liking, caring, trusting, and the public-private dimensions of the relationship will influence the bonds.

The Oxford Supervision Research Group (Beinart & Clohessy, 2017) established that a framework of supervision needs to be established, which they described as a "boundaried relationship." This includes structural boundaries, such as time, place, frequency, and personal-professional boundaries to help the supervisee to feel emotionally contained within the supervisory relationship. The framework also includes the development of a mutually respectful, supportive, and open relationship between supervisor and supervisee.

Bernard and Goodyear (2019) state that developing a positive working alliance is important to produce the following outcomes:

- Internalising the supervisor (Geller, Farber, & Schaffer, 2010)
- Improving the supervisee's therapeutic relationship with their own clients
- Supervisee satisfaction with supervision
- Supervisee's adherence to treatment protocols.

How a supervisory relationship will turn out is likely to be affected by the prior experience of both the supervisee and supervisor. Let me consider an early figure of authority in my own life: My own late father (a photo of whom is on my wall just to the left of my computer screen) was not particularly emotionally warm or empathic. However, amongst his many redeeming features were his calmness, assuredness, spirit of curiosity, playfulness, lack of dogma, and encouragement of debate. I think that these qualities helped me to accept feedback and criticism during my own supervision and to cultivate an ability to learn and develop without feeling crushed when I got things wrong. Contrast this, for example, with one of my supervisees who was devasted by some feedback that I provided her, later telling me that this was triggering something regarding the very difficult relationship that she had with her own father who was very critical. More often, perhaps, the early authority figure will be a schoolteacher (Berman, 2000).

Thinking about what we can learn from attachment theory, Scaife (2001) advocates that the supervision room needs to be a "safe base" where the therapist can openly share their work and the uncertainties that they may have about it. Also, similar to what occurs in a secure attachment, it should ultimately be the responsibility of the supervisor rather than the supervisee to manage the supervisory relationship (Nelson et al., 2001).

When thinking about the supervisory relationship we need to be aware that our style of supervision will need to adapt to the particular learning style of our supervisee and that the "one size fits all" mentality of some supervisors is now outdated (Watkins, 2014). "Some supervisees' worst experience with a supervisor may be another person's best experience and vice versa … A good supervisor, therefore, needs to be flexible enough to adjust their style for each supervisee and, of course, not all people can do this" (Beinart & Clohessy, 2017, p. ix).

Trust and supervisor self-disclosure

As the story that opens this chapter shows, I am a great believer in self-disclosure by the supervisor as a way of enabling the supervisee to feel safe and able to explore their own uncertainties and fears during supervision. I know that not all supervisors will be comfortable with this, but I will explain what I think are the advantages of self-disclosure.

To expand on what I have already mentioned in the last chapter, there is evidence that supervisor self-disclosure enhances the supervisory relationship (Clevinger, Albert, & Raiche, 2019; Knox et al., 2011) and that it functions to ease shame on the part of the supervisee and increase their willingness to self-disclose in turn (Yourman, 2003).

Sharing my clinical mistakes and what I learned from them is a way of normalising the supervisee's sense of shame about disclosing their own mistakes. As I described in Chapter 4, it also shows how we often learn more from what we get wrong than from what we get right.

As well as serving to enhance the supervisory relationship, a study by Ladany and Lehrman-Waterman (1999) found that supervisor self-disclosure aided the repair of ruptures resulting from conflicts and tensions. This has certainly been my own experience.

It should be accepted however that for many supervisors, self-disclosure and openness can be very scary. Whilst we might suppose that more experienced therapists would find it less threatening to be open about their working methods and degree of knowledge, the opposite appears to be the case. Being placed in the role of supervisor can promote a new kind of vulnerability (Boëthius & Ögren, 2014). As EMDR Consultants we are expected to "know the answers" and may feel that our perceived ignorance is no longer acceptable. "Just as we may well underestimate our supervisee's anxiety, it is possible that supervisors may also engage in avoidance behaviors so as to minimise various threats" (Boëthius & Ögren, 2014, p. 354).

I have already mentioned that, according to Bordin (1983), trust is an important element of the supervisory relationship. How does this connect to self-disclosure and openness generally? I cannot do better here than to quote from Scaife: "Building trust takes time and is facilitated by an attitude of openness and authenticity whereby supervisors show evidence of knowing about their own foibles and blind spots and a continuing interest in developing this knowledge further" (Scaife, 2019, p. 87). How to achieve this? Scaife outlines this as follows:

- Not asking the supervisee to do anything that I am not prepared to do first.
- Showing my own work to the supervisee openly either live, with recordings or by modelling.
- Retaining the main focus on the client and drawing everything back to this in the end.
- Always taking a respectful approach to clients and colleagues so that supervisees know that I will not "bad mouth" them behind their backs.
- Not breaking confidences.
- Ensuring that what I say and what I do are congruent.
- If culturally appropriate, discussing how the supervisee can "manage" me should they begin to feel insecure, i.e. talking about the manner in which they might raise issues with me so as not to elicit my defensiveness.
- Making sure that my challenges are specific and related to the work.
- Considering whether it would be helpful to comment on areas where I am unsure, don't know or feel I have made an error, and talking about how to take the work forward.
- Where relevant, talking about my own training experiences and how I may differ now from then.
- Not showing off my knowledge in the service of my own ego.
- Being prepared to take a position of authority and give instructions where client or supervisee safety is at issue.
- Letting supervisees know that they will not be allowed to act outside the boundaries that keep the system safe.
- Considering sharing some personal information in a way that I might not with clients – to allow me as a human being to show through my professional bearing.
- Showing interest in the supervisee as a person as well as a professional.
- Noticing the supervisee's knowledge and skills.

(Scaife, 2019, pp. 99–100)

Supervisee self-disclosure

Some readers may be thinking, "this section of the book is rather wishy-washy and there should be more focus on how to ensure that our supervisees are actually doing EMDR right!" Well, we cannot achieve this unless our supervisees feel safe enough to disclose their mistakes.

Ladany et al. (1996) found that 97% of supervisees had withheld information from their supervisors and, in 50% of cases, supervisees said they were not disclosing their mistakes due to a poor alliance with the supervisor.

There are also cultural factors at play here. For example, Wu (2012) compared Asian international students with home-based American students. The Asian students were more likely to be reluctant to self-disclose, would overvalue the supervisor's opinions, and behave passively towards more senior people. In a study by Yourman and Farber (1996) about 40% of supervisees said that they had "omitted describing details of my work that I have felt were clinical errors" at one time or another and I have to confess to being one of that 40% myself.

This is a serious problem because, as Bernard and Goodyear (2019) point out, supervisees are putting their clients at risk when they fail to disclose relevant information about them and their treatment. Supervisees are also putting limitations on what they can learn in supervision. Farrell (2020) suggested the following reasons why EMDR supervisees may fail to disclose information about their therapy:

1   Believe that the EMDR clinical supervisor would judge the information to be "irrelevant"
2   That they might experience negative feelings, including shame, disapproval, and disappointment
3   Perceived differences in cultural background and cultural competency
4   Source of conflict between therapy approaches
5   Concern over clinical mistakes and potential errors of judgment
6   Disclosing vulnerability
7   Outcome focussed – therefore wishing to ensure positive evaluation
(Farrell, 2020, slide 12)

Farrell's last point clearly relates to the Evaluating functions of supervision which will be covered in the next chapter. There is undoubtedly a tension here for the supervisee in terms of balancing learning, which will require disclosure, with their desire to receive a positive evaluation. This tension may, they feel, necessitate keeping information about their therapy sessions under wraps (Hess, 2008).

Much of what may be difficult for supervisees to disclose is their perception that they have made a mistake during therapy. In such situations, I find it helpful to take what the supervisee may perceive as a "disaster" and reframe it as "new information" that will help the therapist to respond to their client in a more therapeutic way. One of my supervisees told me, "I have found it helpful how you talk about your own mistakes, or when things haven't gone according to plan, as this helps me with feeling able to accept my own mistakes and to not put too much pressure on myself to have to get it 'right' all the time."

It is also important to mention the role of shame in preventing disclosure by supervisees (Farrell's second point). Hahn (2001) addresses the function of shame in the development of attachment to caregivers and how this is projected into the supervisory relationship. When shame is activated, supervisees have three options:

- They can acknowledge to themselves that they are experiencing shame and silently struggle to maintain their composure.
- They can acknowledge to their supervisor that they feel inadequate and incompetent and share their belief that they will be condemned for their incompetence. Most supervisees will find this impossible to admit.
- They can react to the shame to protect themselves from their overwhelming and disorganizing experience.

The third of these is the most likely outcome. Nathanson (1994) has identified four common reactions to shame which, according to Hahn, are likely protective reactions to occur in the supervision session:

- withdrawal
- avoidance
- attack on self
- attack on others

Hahn says that, irrespective of how shame is triggered and manifested, supervisors should avoid the temptation of confronting shameful reactions or prematurely referring supervisees for personal therapy. "Supervisor self-disclosure and normalization of treatment hurdles can help supervisees feel competent relative to their level of training" (p. 280).

The parallel process

I have already referred to the parallel process in Chapter 3 when outlining the Seven-Eyed model of supervision (Hawkins, 1985; Hawkins & McMahon, 2020). A parallel process (Doehrman, 1976; McNeill & Worthen, 1989) may be occurring in which the supervisory relationship is manifesting similar relationship dynamics to those in the therapeutic relationship. For example, a particular client may be very dependent on the therapist which may be reflected in the therapist appearing to be dependent on the supervisor when discussing a particular client. Or a client whose Negative Cognition (NC) is "I'm not good enough" may manifest in the parallel process as the therapist feeling "I'm not a good enough therapist." What happens in the therapy room may be re-enacted in supervision (Bernard & Goodyear, 2019) and, conversely, what happens in supervision may be re-enacted in the therapy room (Frawley-O'Dea & Sarnat, 2001).

I recall a supervisee, who usually presented their clients to me in a clear and succinct way. She appeared confused and hesitant when presenting a particular client to the point where I myself felt muddled and anchorless. When I reflected this back to my supervisee, it helped her to realise that there were issues in her relationship with her client that she had not previously recognised and that this was getting in the way of her being able to help her client with EMDR therapy.

It has been pointed out however that the notion of the parallel process creates a risk of creating an assumption that all issues between supervisor and supervisee are a reflection of the therapeutic relationship. Focusing on this too much may lead to avoidance of addressing conflicts in the supervisory relationship itself (Berman, 2000; Scaife, 2019).

Telling my story

I am sure that most readers of this book will have encountered the client who resists the format of questions and answers that is usually involved during History Taking and insists on "telling my story." Often one has to allow the client to tell the story before asking any specific questions and, in most cases, many of the therapist's standard questions will have been answered during the telling of the story. The same will sometimes occur in supervision. Whilst we may want to focus on the Supervision Question and a specific dialogue around this focus, there will be some cases presented by supervisees, often where high levels of therapist emotion are involved, where we need to be sensitive to our supervisee and just allow them to "tell the story." Telling the story is sometimes a way of getting to a particularly obscure Supervision Question.

Obviously, if this happens at every supervision session with every client it is something that would need to be addressed. But if it occurs occasionally with a particular client, the supervisor should accept that this is an important aspect of the Enabling function of supervision.

On one occasion, after being asked for their Supervision Question, my supervisee said, "just validation, really." On another occasion, the response was "I know the answer to my question. I just think that if I talk about it, I'm more likely to do it." In my view, these are legitimate "questions" and point to the fact that, with this particular client, it is the enabling role that we need to inhabit.

The power relationship

We have already talked about shame and self-disclosure in supervision. Coupled with that is the Evaluating aspect of supervision (to be covered in the next chapter) which clearly leads to a significant imbalance of power in the supervisory relationship. If we deny that there is a power differential in supervision, we are deluding ourselves and will actually make this more of a problem than it needs to be. "The supervisor's greater power can be problematic if the supervisor is oblivious to it, abuses it, or (more typically) has difficulty using it comfortably" (Bernard & Goodyear, 2019, p. 110).

Clearly supervisor power can be abused by the supervisor, for example, pathologising supervisees and attempting to give them therapy instead of supervision, selectively focusing on their limitations, verbally attacking supervisees, insistence on adherence to the supervisor's approach or even unwanted sexual advances (Porter & Vasquez, 1997). But power can be used in a positive way to protect the client and enhance the supervisee's learning (Bernard & Goodyear, 2019).

Trainees will not practise EMDR without supervision

Much of this chapter, whilst being relevant to EMDR supervision, has not been specifically about EMDR supervision. However, this final section addresses a specific issue pertaining to EMDR that is particularly relevant to the Enabling function of supervision. One of the most important aspects of this function is to provide the necessary support to trainees who have just embarked on their training in EMDR.

The experience of those trained in EMDR is that supervision is necessary in order for them to continue to use EMDR beyond their basic training (Dodaj & Dodaj, 2021). In a study in the USA, EMDR therapists regarded ongoing supervision as the most important factor for the continued use of EMDR and 40% of respondents ranked its importance high on their lists (Grimmett & Galvin, 2015). Kerr (2009) carried out a qualitative study to look at the reasons why those trained in EMDR were not integrating it into their practice. One of her interviews went as follows:

- I: So have you done any EMDR yet?
- P: No
- I: So what do you think has stopped you?
- P: I think primarily, not being able to access supervision (p. 89)

All of the respondents identified further training and development needs following the EMDR training including ... most importantly, supervision (p. 59).

My own experience from my work as a trainer is that those individuals who have attended my Part 1 training and have been unable to access EMDR supervision, for whatever reason, are unlikely to have actually started using EMDR with their clients. It is therefore likely that trainees will simply not use EMDR after they have been trained if they have not received specific supervision in EMDR.

Very often, in the supervision of therapists who have only recently trained in EMDR or are still undergoing their training, the Supervision Question is usually, "Is this client suitable for EMDR?" The only thing I need to say as their supervisor, is "yeah, great! Go for it!" Some supervisees are quite phobic of commencing EMDR Phase 4 processing. As I have already mentioned in Chapter 3, in such situations I will ask the Flashforward (Logie & De Jongh, 2014) question: "what's the worst thing that could happen if you started processing now?"

Conclusion

This chapter has covered a vital aspect of EMDR supervision, the Enabling function. Without a sound supervisory relationship, grounded in trust and acceptance, supervisees will be unable to share their uncertainties and admit their mistakes. And without this, supervisees are unlikely to be able to use supervision to enhance their practice as EMDR therapists.

Baier, A. L., Kline, A. C., & Feeny, N. C. (2020). Therapeutic alliance as a mediator of change: A systematic review and evaluation of research. *Clinical Psychology Review, 82*, 101921.

Beinart, H., & Clohessy, S. (2017). *Effective supervisory relationships. Best evidence and practice.* Chichester, UK: Wiley.

Berman, E. (2000). Psychanalytic supervision: The intersubjective development. *International Journal of Psychoanalysis, 81*, 273–290.

Bernard, J. M., & Goodyear, R. K. (2019). *Fundimentals of clinical supervision* (6th ed.). New York, NY: Pearson.

Boëthius, S., & Ögren, M. (2014). Developing understanding in supervision. In C. Watkins & D. Milne (Eds.), *The Wiley international handbook of clinical supervision* (pp. 342–363). Chichester, West Sussex: Wiley.

Booth, P. B., & Jernberg, A. M. (2010). *Theraplay: Helping parents and children build better relationships through attachment-based play.* San Francisco, CA: John Wiley & Sons.

Bordin, E. S. (1983). A working alliance based model of supervision. *The Counseling Psychologist, 11*(1), 35–42.

Clevinger, K., Albert, E., & Raiche, E. (2019). Supervisor self-disclosure: Supervisees' perceptions of positive supervision experiences. *Training and Education in Professional Psychology, 13*(3), 222.

Dodaj, A., & Dodaj, A. (2021). Experience of an EMDR practitioner in EMDR education: Case report. *Psychiatria Danubina, 33*(Suppl 1), 100–102.

Doehrman, M. J. G. (1976). Parallel processes in supervision and psychotherapy. *Bulletin of the Meninger Clinic, 40*, 9–104.

Farrell, D. (2020). *Advanced clinical supervision and consultation skills in enhancing competency in EMDR therapy.* EMDR Lebanon Association.

Frawley-O'Dea, M. G., & Sarnat, J. E. (2001). *The supervisory relationship: A contemporary psychodynamic approach.* New York: Guilford Press.

Geller, J. D., Farber, B. A., & Schaffer, C. E. (2010). Representations of the supervisory dialogue and the development of psychotherapists. *Psychotherapy: Theory, Research, Practice, Training, 47*(2), 211.

Grimmett, J., & Galvin, M. (2015). Clinician experiences with EMDR: Factors influencing continued use. *Journal of EMDR Practice and Research, 9*(1), 3–16.

Hahn, W. K. (2001). The experience of shame in psychotherapy supervision. *Psychotherapy: Theory, Research, Practice, Training, 38*(3), 272–282.

Hawkins, P. (1985). Humanistic psychotherapy supervision: A conceptual framework. *Self & Society*, *13*(2), 69–76.

Hawkins, P., & McMahon, A. (2020). *Supervision in the helping professions* (5th ed.). London: Open University Press.

Hess, A. K. (2008). Psychotherapy supervision: A conceptual review. In K. D. Hess, & T. H. Hess (Eds.), *Psychotherapy supervision: Theory, research, and practice* (pp. 3–22). Hoboken, NJ: Wiley.

Kerr, C. (2009). *Why do some EMDR trained therapists choose not to integrate this therapy into their practice to work with PTSD?* (MSC thesis), University of Chester.

Knox, S., Edwards, L. M., Hess, S. A., & Hill, C. E. (2011). Supervisor self-disclosure: Supervisees' experiences and perspectives. *Psychotherapy*, *48*(4), 336.

Ladany, N., & Lehrman-Waterman, D. (1999). The content and frequency of supervisor self-disclosure and their relationship to supervisor style and supervisory working alliance. *Counselor Education and Supervision*, *38*, 143–160.

Ladany, N., Hill, C. E., Corbett, M. M., & Nutt, E. A. (1996). Nature, extent, and importance of what psychotherapy trainees do not disclose to their supervisors. *Journal of Counseling Psychology*, *43*(1), 10.

Lesser, R. M. (1983). Supervision: Illusions, anxieties, and questions. *Contemporary Psychoanalysis*, *19*, 120–129.

Logie, R., & De Jongh, A. (2014). The "Flashforward procedure": Confronting the catastrophe. *Journal of EMDR Practice and Research*, *8*(1), 25–32.

McNeill, B. W., & Worthen, V. (1989). The parallel process in psychotherapy supervision. *Professional Psychology: Research and Practice*, *20*(5), 329.

Nathanson, D. L. (1994). *Shame and pride: Affect, sex, and the birth of the self*. New York: WW Norton & Company.

Nelson, M. L., Gray, L. A., Friedlander, M. L., Ladany, N., & Walker, J. A. (2001). Toward relationship-centered supervision: Reply to Veach (2001) and Ellis (2001). *Journal of Counseling Psychology*, *48*, 407–409.

Porter, N., & Vasquez, M. (1997). Covision: Feminist supervision, process, and collaboration. In J. Worell, & N. G. Johnson (Eds.), *Shaping the future of feminist psychology* (pp. 155–171). Washington, DC: American Psychological Association.

Proctor, B. (1988). Supervision: a co-operative exercise in accountability. In M. Marken, & M. Payne (Eds.), *Enabling and ensuring*. Leicester: National Youth Bureau and Council for Education and Training in Youth and Community Work.

Roth, A. D., & Pilling, S. (2008). Using an evidence-based methodology to identify the competences required to deliver effective cognitive and behavioural therapy for depression and anxiety disorders. *Behavioural and Cognitive Psychotherapy*, *36*(2), 129–147.

Scaife, J. (2001). *Supervising the reflective practitioner: an essential guide to theory and practice*. Hove, East Sussex: Routledge.

Scaife, J. (2019). *Supervision in clinical practice: a practitioner's guide* (3rd ed.). Milton Park, Abingdon, Oxon: Routledge.

Watkins, C. E. (2014). The supervisory alliance: A half century of theory, practice, and research in critical perspective. *American Journal of Psychotherapy*, *68*(1), 19–55.

Wu, Y.-C. (2012). *Contributing factors for supervisory relationships, cultural discussions, and acculturation process in supervision with Asian international counseling trainees: cognitive style, theoretical orientation, and supervisory style.* PhD thesis, University of Georgia.

Yourman, D. (2003). Trainee disclosure in psychotherapy supervision: The impact of shame. *Journal of Clinical Psychology, 59*(5), 601–609.

Yourman, D., & Farber, B. (1996). Nondisclosure and distortion in psychotherapy supervison. *Psychotherapy: Theory, Research, Practice, Training, 33*(4), 567.

Chapter 6

The "Evaluating" function
Ensuring good practice and adherence to the protocol

- Why do we need a system of accreditation?
- EMDR Europe accreditation system
- EMDR Europe Competency Framework
- How to evaluate competency
- Measuring competency
- "Consultant hopping"
- Giving feedback
- Supervisees who do not wish to pursue accreditation
- Ensuring ethical practice

Emily and the horse

My daughter Emily is a farm vet. When she was training at Bristol University, she was required to carry out a procedure on a horse and was observed by one of her tutors to check whether she was carrying out the procedure according to the approved protocol. The horse had to be restrained whilst Emily injected it in the leg. There were several things that Emily was required to do before the injection. However, the horse was becoming increasingly agitated and Emily knew that, if she did not inject quickly, the horse would become out of control and she would be unable to safely administer the injection. She therefore skipped one part of the procedure and jabbed the needle into the horse and injected it safely.

When the procedure had been completed, Emily's tutor asked her if she could state what the correct procedure was. Emily correctly outlined the procedure. Her tutor asked her therefore why she had omitted one part of the procedure. Emily explained that if she had done it according to the book, there was a distinct risk that the horse's agitation would have made it impossible for her to give the injection. The tutor told her that she was absolutely right and awarded her full marks for the assessment.

The moral of this story, if it hasn't become obvious already, is that it is important to know what the protocol is. There are times when you need to

DOI: 10.4324/9781003214588-7

deviate from the protocol, but you should do so knowingly and be able to give a rational justification for doing so.

The previous two chapters have covered the Educating and Enabling functions of supervision. Always in the background, in relation to clinical supervision, even when these two functions are in operation, is the fact that, as supervisors, we are evaluating the competence of our supervisees. This chapter will cover this area and particularly as it applies to the supervision of EMDR therapists.

Why do we need a system of accreditation?

Firstly, it should be pointed out that the basic seven to eight-day training in EMDR does not include an element of evaluation of the trainee. At the end of each part of the training, the trainee receives a certificate of attendance. This shows that they have attended the training but does not state that they have attained any particular level of competence. It is only during the next stage in their training, whilst receiving supervision during the process of accreditation as an EMDR Practitioner, that any actual evaluation of the supervisee's abilities takes place.

In her Consultant's trainings in the UK, Sandi Richman (Richman, 2021) outlines why accreditation as an EMDR therapist is important. In the acquisition and development of skills and knowledge, an EMDR clinician moves from being an EMDR novice to hopefully achieving a high level of EMDR proficiency and expertise. One of the important ways of achieving this is through accreditation. According to Richman, the benefits of accreditation are that it:

• maximises the teaching and learning experience of EMDR training
• ensures ethically sound and robust EMDR clinical practice
• enhances EMDR treatment fidelity
• monitors and maximises client protection
• enhances quality control
• greatly assists towards research fidelity
• defines a minimum standard of practice across all of Europe

EMDR Europe accreditation system

As mentioned in the Introduction, this book is, of necessity, pitched mainly at readers from Europe. It is therefore the EMDR Europe accreditation system that this chapter will be based upon.

It should be noted that the system of accreditation in Europe is under constant review and readers of this book should always check the website of their relevant EMDR association in order to ascertain the up-to-date details regarding the current requirements and specifications for accreditation.

At the time of writing, we have the following levels of accreditation in EMDR Europe:

- Practitioner
- Consultant (supervisor)
- Facilitator
- Trainer

This chapter will focus mainly on the first of these categories – Practitioner accreditation. Consultant accreditation will be covered in Chapter 12 whilst Chapter 11 will cover the role of the Facilitator.

There are a number of criteria that need to be satisfied in order to become accredited as an EMDR Europe Practitioner and these can be found on the website of each national EMDR association. As far as EMDR supervisors are concerned, the following criteria are those that we need to focus on: The applicant needs to have:

- treated a minimum of 25 clients (minimum of 50 sessions) since commencement of their basic EMDR training, all of whom the supervisee has discussed with their supervisor
- received a minimum of 20 hours of supervision from an EMDR Europe accredited Consultant (including the 10 hours received during training)
- demonstrated competency in all parts of the competency framework which has included the supervisor directly witnessing the supervisee's EMDR work on video or in vivo

It is the last of these that is, in fact, the most important. To illustrate this, I often tell my own trainees and supervisees the story of my own experience when I was at this stage of my development as an EMDR therapist. After the required minimum of 20 hours of supervision, I asked my supervisor if he would now sign me off and approve my accreditation as a Practitioner. I don't recall his exact words, but it will have been something along these lines: "Well Robin, actually I don't think you are quite ready yet. There are still some things that we need to work on. I need to be sure you are really sticking to the protocol and I am not yet satisfied that you are." In retrospect, I am sure that he was right. The bottom line in terms of accreditation is that the supervisor needs to be certain that the supervisee really has the EMDR Standard Protocol under their belt and is able to use EMDR competently.

EMDR Europe competency framework

As EMDR supervisors, we should always be cognisant of the competency framework in the country in which we operate. This should always be in the back of our mind when we are thinking about the Evaluating function of supervision. The EMDR Europe Competency Framework is reproduced in Appendix 3.

How to evaluate competency

So how, as an EMDR Consultant, should we go about assessing the extent to which our supervisees are competent in relation to the criteria stated above?

Firstly, where do we get our information from? Chapter 10 will be devoted to reviewing the different media for observing our supervisees' work and the various pros and cons of each in relation to each of the functions of supervision. Bernard and Goodyear (2019) outline the different media by which we can receive data regarding our supervisee's work as follows:

- Reporting back on therapy sessions
- Written transcripts of sessions
- Live supervision
- Viewing videos of sessions
- Roleplay

It is the first of these (reporting back on therapy sessions) that will usually form the bulk of the information that supervisor will have at their disposal when evaluating the extent to which the Competency Framework criteria are being met. It is important, for the purposes of evaluation, and for other reasons which I will outline, that we keep careful contemporaneous notes as we supervise our colleagues. We need to ensure that we have been informed about each of the clients that have been listed on the accreditation application in order to "sign them off." To this effect, I find it useful to always ask for the initials of the client when they are being presented and also to make a note if this client has previously been presented by my supervisee.

If I am observing a therapy session ("live supervision") or a video I will also keep detailed notes of what I have observed. In order to facilitate my subsequent feedback to my supervisee I will place an asterisk in the margin of my notes if I spot a violation of the Standard Protocol which I may wish to discuss with my supervisee. I also place a tick in the margin when there is particular aspect of what I have observed that I wish to commend my supervisee on. These notes should form the basis of the supervisor's evaluation.

It should also be mentioned that keeping notes may be important for legal reasons if, for example, a complaint is made about the supervisee or if their client is to give evidence in court.

Measuring competency

How do we evaluate whether our supervisee is "competent" and suitable for Practitioner accreditation, based upon what we have observed of their practice and have been told in supervision? In EMDR we have the advantage of having a clear list of desired competencies, but how do we ascertain that these competencies have been attained?

Recently, EMDR Europe has introduced the "algorithm" version of the accreditation form. Instead of writing a short report in relation to each set of competencies, Consultants can opt to rate each individual competency on the following scale:

- Novice (score = 1)
- Intermediate (score = 2)
- Competent (score = 3)
- Advanced (score = 4)

There are 58 competencies listed and if a therapist was scored as "competent" on all 58 competencies, they would achieve a score of 174 which is the minimum score required for accreditation purposes. Obviously, if they were scored as "advanced" on some competencies they could still achieve a score of 174 or more whilst only being rated as "intermediate" on other competencies. However, in order to be accredited, a therapist should be rated as at least "competent" on all 58 competencies. If they are any less than competent on any competency, they are clearly not yet ready to apply for accreditation.

At present, Consultants can opt to use either the traditional narrative form or the newer algorithm form. I would suggest, however, that even when using the narrative form, Consultants should bear in mind that they should not be approving a therapist for Practitioner accreditation unless they are satisfied that they have achieved a level of competence on all 58 competencies.

It should also be accepted that the evaluation of competency does not need to be a one-way process and, if the supervisor and supervisee can collaborate on this process, it can lead to a more satisfactory and dynamic supervisory relationship. "Self-assessment is at the heart of developing and maintaining competence … as an individual must identify areas of strength and weakness to establish priorities and to commit to learning strategies to ensure competent practice" (Falender & Shafranske, 2007, p. 236). Borders and Brown (2005) suggest that the supervisee should understand from the beginning that they will be expected to complete a self-evaluation at the end of the supervisory experience. Requiring supervisees to provide a final narrative, self-reflective report helps them to review the supervision experience in its entirety, and synthesize the various aspects of their growth process. Woolliscroft (2021) suggests that EMDR therapists are asked to write the first draft of their own accreditation application as a way of helping them to reflect on their progress in relation to their EMDR practice. "Having supervisees identify their own performance deficiencies prior to their supervisor's evaluation is intended to minimize resistance from trainees" (Sobell et al., 2008, p. 152).

"Consultant hopping"

There is a phenomenon amongst EMDR therapists (and for other therapies too, I have no doubt) of some supervisees transferring to different Consultants in the hope that they may get a more favourable response regarding their application for accreditation. It is for this reason, that all Consultants should be careful to ask any new supervisee about their previous EMDR supervisor and their reasons for changing supervisor. Fortunately, the supervisor is obliged to "sign off" all the cases presented for accreditation and this therefore gives the supervisor a legitimate reason to contact the previous supervisor to compare notes and to check whether there had been any problems in relation to the previous supervision. However, the previous Consultant should not just be asked how many clients have been supervised but also about their views on the supervisee's competency.

Giving feedback

One of the difficulties that I have had when writing this book has been in relation to what to put where. For example, giving feedback to your supervisee is not just a topic that relates to the Evaluating function of supervision. It also relates very much to the Educating function, but on balance this seems to be the most appropriate place to discuss it.

Firstly, let us differentiate "formative feedback" from "summative feedback" which is also relevant to my dilemma as to whether to put this section in this chapter or in the chapter regarding the Educating function of supervision. "Formative feedback" describes the everyday corrective feedback which should, in fact, occur at every supervision session as the supervisor is commenting on the cases being presented and teaching as she goes along. In contrast, "summative feedback" relates to telling the supervisee whether their performance has reached the standard required for accreditation, sometimes referred to as the "gate-keeping" function of supervision (Milne, 2018). "Formative feedback is focussed on development and progress whereas summative feedback focusses on outcomes" (Beinart & Clohessy, 2017, p. 92).

It appears that when formative feedback is ongoing and is managed effectively, the Evaluating role of giving summative feedback can seem less daunting (Beinart, 2002). For some reason, I am reminded of the difference between a marriage where there are daily niggles and stuff gets sorted out in the relationship from day to day compared with the marriage where everything goes too smoothly but there is then an annual general bust up. "Summative assessment most helpfully emerges out of formative assessment so that there are no surprises ..." (Scaife, 2019, p. 271).

Formative feedback

So let us start by thinking more about formative feedback. Firstly the supervisory relationship needs to have the right atmosphere to enable this to happen. Bernard and Goodyear (2019) quote Ekstein and Wallerstein (1972) who say that when the context of supervision is favourable, the supervisee stops asking, "How can I avoid criticism?" and starts asking, "How can I make the most of this supervision time?"

Many supervisors tend to make the mistake of avoiding making constructive criticism (Hoffman et al., 2005). As therapists we are in the business of developing supportive, caring and non-critical relationships with our clients. It is therefore difficult for many of us, when becoming supervisors, to make the transition to adding an evaluative and, frankly, "critical" element to our relationship with our supervisees. Nelson et al. (2008) refer to "gate-keeping anxiety" whilst Brown and Marzillier (1993) warn against the "cult of the positive." As Fleming et al. (2007) ask, "might peer supervision become devoid of critical reflection, mutate into backslapping and become part of what has been called the 'tyranny of niceness'?"

Ladany and Melincoff (1999) found that 98% of their sample of supervisors withheld feedback from their supervisees. They gave reasons such as preferring to avoid confrontation, concerns about the negative impact on the supervisees, or a belief that supervisees will learn themselves when they are developmentally ready.

Once we have accepted that we need to give feedback to our supervisees which may, at times, be difficult for them to accept, what is the most effective way of doing this?

Let us start by learning from one of my worst mistakes: I once told a supervisee that, in the way that she related to her client on the video, she appeared "cold." She was extremely upset by this feedback. So where did I go wrong? Describing my supervisee as "cold" left her with no suggestion of how she might change or move forward. It would have been more helpful to her had I been specific about which aspects of her behaviour towards her client seemed "cold" in order that she could then think about how she might be able to change her behaviour. Interestingly, this had resonance for me as it reminded me of my very first placement as a trainee clinical psychologist working in a day hospital. At that time my supervisor told me that the staff at the hospital perceived me as being rather aloof and off-hand with them. This feedback surprised me. And my supervisor was, in turn, surprised when I told her that I was probably behaving this way due to my own anxiety.

So, how should I have given feedback to my supervisee? Hattie and Timperley (2007) distinguished four levels of feedback:

- feedback about the *task*
- feedback about the *processing* or strategies used to do the task
- feedback about *self-regulation* related to the task (self-evaluation and self-confidence)
- feedback about the trainee as a *person*

They found that feedback from the first two (*task* and *processing*) are the most effective in producing change, while the other two can often fail to produce the desired effect. Feedback about the person whether positive or negative (for example, "You are very intelligent/disorganized") is not regarded as helpful for two reasons. Firstly, it does not contain information that can be used to improve learning. Secondly, such feedback can give the impression that the abilities highlighted reflect unchangeable traits (Brookhart, 2017) and thus achievement on this aspect is beyond the trainees' control. Giving feedback about trainees' abilities, even praise, can lead to a significant decrease in performance.

Hawkins and McMahon (2020) use the mnemonic CORBS (Clear, Owned, Regular, Balanced, and Specific) to summarise how to give helpful feedback:

- *Clear:* Be clear about the feedback. Don't be vague.
- *Owned:* The feedback is your own perception and not the ultimate truth. (We need to acknowledge, however, that in EMDR supervision, if the feedback relates to the Standard Protocol, we may need to be more emphatic and tell our supervisees that "this is what the protocol is" and explain why things are done in this way, if possible, explaining the rationale in terms of the AIP model.)
- *Regular:* Give feedback regularly and as close as possible to the event.
- *Balanced:* Provide positive as well as negative feedback. The positive feedback does not need to occur every time there is negative feedback, but it should be balanced over time. (However, see discussion of the "feedback sandwich" below.)
- *Specific:* Describe the specific behaviour that the supervisee may be able to change. This will give them some direction and make it less likely that they respond with hurt and anger.

To elaborate on the notion of being "balanced," Dohrenwend (2002) coined the term "feedback sandwich" to describe a technique of preceding any negative feedback with some positive feedback and then following it up with more positive feedback. This can be particularly useful with someone who is just starting out as an EMDR therapist or where the particular supervisory relationship is quite new. James (2015) says that the feedback sandwich is outdated and suggests replacing it with something more subtle in which the supervisee is helped to find their own answers. In my own experience, however, supervisees just want me to get on with it and tell them straight. I have had supervisees saying to me, "OK, there's no need to give me the shit sandwich [as it is more colloquially known]. Just crack on and tell me what I've done wrong!"

Summative feedback

As stated above, when it gets to the point of summative feedback (telling your supervisee whether you believe they are ready for accreditation) there should be few surprises if the formative feedback has been effective.

So there comes a crunch point when it is time for the supervisor and supervisee to confront the question as to whether the supervisee is ready to apply for accreditation. Interestingly this might be prompted either by the supervisee or by the supervisor. In an ideal situation (which rarely happens!) they will both come to this conclusion simultaneously. More often it is the supervisee who pops the question to the supervisor, "do you think I am ready for accreditation yet?" Sometimes it is the supervisor who broaches the subject, and, on some occasions, the supervisee seems surprised that the supervisor is suggesting that they are ready for accreditation. (In my experience, these are usually the more modest but also the more competent supervisees.)

The biggest problem to address here, related to the last point I made, is the supervisee who believes that they are ready for accreditation when the supervisor believes that they are not ready. Described as the "Dunning-Kruger effect," there is tendency of people with lower ability in a specific area to give overly positive assessments of their own ability and to greatly overestimate their competence or to see themselves as more skilled than they actually are (Dunning, 2011). Even when the supervisor has been competently offering formative feedback, some supervisees will not really be hearing this, and it may come as a shock to them when their supervisor tells them that they are not yet ready for accreditation. In some cases, the issue is that the supervisee is more motivated to achieve accreditation than to actually learn and develop their practice during the course of supervision. Their focus will therefore be more on demonstrating their ability to their supervisor than to learn from them (Stoltenberg et al., 2014).

With such supervisees it will be necessary to be very specific and explicit about the areas on which they still need to develop competence. Making reference, for example, to the EMDR Europe Competency Framework can be useful here. The supervisor can go through the form with the supervisee, point by point, explaining how and why they are not yet competent in particular areas. It is then important for the supervisor to explain how each area can be worked on in order for the supervisee to achieve competence. Whilst it is necessary for the supervisor to show their authority in such a situation, they also need to accept that such a situation can expose deep feelings of shame for the supervisee. This may be mitigated to a certain extent by the supervisor modelling their own humility, perhaps by telling the supervisee about a time when they, themselves, were in such a situation (Beinart & Clohessy, 2017). In my case, I have plenty to choose from, the most notable one being the time when I had the viva for my Doctor of Clinical Psychology thesis and was told by the panel that it was not adequate and that I should resubmit it in 12 months' time.

In Chapter 8, I will go into more detail about how to manage problems in the supervisory relationship which will often emerge at this stage where we are providing summative feedback to inform our supervisees that they are not yet ready for accreditation.

Supervisees who do not wish to pursue accreditation

In the UK, less than 20% of those who train in EMDR subsequently become accredited (Farrell, 2020). There will be a number of reasons for this. In a study by Farrell and Keenan (2013) it was more common for counsellors (48%) and psychotherapists (70%) to be accredited than for, for example, mental health nurses (23%), social workers (21%), or psychologists (36%). They note that those in private practice are more likely to pursue accreditation and one would assume that this is because accreditation would enhance their professional development more. By contrast those employed in statutory agencies are less likely to become accredited. "Several mental health nurses responded that they considered accreditation in EMDR to gain them 'no added value' in terms of their employment or career development. In addition, several participants described case examples where employers asked them to merely be EMDR trained rather than accredited" (p. 10).

If we have a supervisee who does not wish to seek accreditation, how should we approach this with them? I believe that it is useful to explain the importance of accreditation to our supervisees not just as an extra qualification but also to explain how the actual process of accreditation, including viewing of videos and systematic reference to the EMDR Europe Competency Framework can enhance their development as an EMDR therapist even if they do not need the piece of paper at the end of this process. However, I would be loath to refuse to supervise someone because they did not wish to seek accreditation, as this would potentially mean that they would receive no supervision at all for their EMDR practice.

Ensuring ethical practice

Whether or not our supervisee wishes to become accredited we have an additional Evaluating function as EMDR supervisors – to ensure that our supervisees are practising safely and ethically. To be honest none of the issues in this section are specific to EMDR and are, in fact, relevant to anyone practising as a psychological therapist. However, I am including this section for the sake of completeness and to ensure that those who provide EMDR supervision are fully aware of these issues.

We should bear in mind that, in order to train as an EMDR therapist, an individual must be accredited in their core profession with a professional body such as the British Association for Counselling and Psychotherapy (BACP) or the Health and Care Professions Council (HCPC). Ultimately it will be to the accrediting body of their core profession that any complaints about their practice would be made. As EMDR supervisors we are acting usually in a capacity of consultancy and are not legally responsible for our supervisee's practice. However, it would be our duty to address any issues that have come to our attention regarding our supervisee's fitness to practise and, if necessary, report this to their accrediting professional organisation.

Bernard and Goodyear (2019) refer to "problems of professional competence" (PPC) and use the definition of Shen-Miller et al. (2015): "PPC include difficulty in acquiring or maintaining developmentally appropriate levels of skill, functioning, attitudes, and/or ethical, professional or foundational domains in one or more settings" (p. 162).

Any issues should of course be first raised with the supervisee. But supervisors must accept that, if things cannot be satisfactorily resolved, they may need to report their concerns to the supervisee's employer or professional organisation (Scaife, 2019).

Please note the comments that have already been made in relation to record-keeping in Chapter 2. If a complaint is made about a supervisee, it may be necessary for the supervisor to disclose their own supervision notes or records.

For a more details discussion of the ethical dilemmas that may arise during supervision, I refer you to an excellent chapter on this topic in Scaife (2019).

Conclusion

The Evaluative function of EMDR supervision relates mainly to the process of accreditation. However, the feedback that we give to our supervisees about their practice should be an ongoing process throughout supervision. If this is achieved successfully it is less likely that there will be a major disruption to the supervisory relationship when the time comes to discuss whether a supervisee is ready for accreditation.

Beinart, H. (2002). *An exploration of the factors which predict the quality of the relationship in clinical supervision.* UK: Open University.

Beinart, H., & Clohessy, S. (2017). *Effective supervisory relationships. Best evidence and practice.* Chichester, UK: Wiley.

Bernard, J. M., & Goodyear, R. K. (2019). *Fundamentals of clinical supervision* (6th ed.). New York, NY: Pearson.

Borders, L. D., & Brown, L. L. (2005). *The new handbook of counseling supervision.*

Brookhart, S. M. (2017). *How to give effective feedback to your students: ASCD.*

Brown, B., & Marzillier, J. (1993). *The evaluation of clinical competence: Report on the proceedings of Joint CUCPTC and the CORIC workshop held at Grasmere, Cumbria.* Grasmere, Cumbria: CUCPTC & CORIC.

Dohrenwend, A. (2002). Serving up the feedback sandwich. *Family Practice Management, 9*(10), 43.

Dunning, D. (2011). The Dunning–Kruger effect: On being ignorant of one's own ignorance. In *Advances in experimental social psychology* (Vol. 44, pp. 247–296): Elsevier.

Ekstein, R., & Wallerstein, R. S. (1972). *The teaching and learning of psychotherapy* (2nd ed.). New York, NY: International Universities Press.

Falender, C. A., & Shafranske, E. P. (2007). Competence in competency-based supervision practice: Construct and application. *Professional Psychology: Research and Practice*, *38*(3), 232.

Farrell, D. (2020). *Advanced clinical supervision and consultation skills in enhancing competency in EMDR therapy*. EMDR Lebanon Association.

Farrell, D., & Keenan, P. (2013). Participants' experiences of EMDR training in the United Kingdom and Ireland. *Journal of EMDR Practice and Research*, *7*(1), 2–16.

Fleming, I., Gone, R., Diver, A., & Fowler, B. (2007). Risk supervision in Rochdale. *Clinical Psychology Forum*, *176* 22–25.

Hattie, J., & Timperley, H. (2007). The power of feedback. *Review of Educational Research*, *77*(1), 81–112.

Hawkins, P., & McMahon, A. (2020). *Supervision in the helping professions* (5th ed.). London: Open University Press.

Hoffman, M. A., Hill, C. E., Holmes, S. E., & Freitas, G. F. (2005). Supervisor perspective on the process and outcome of gfiving easy, difficult, or no feedback to supervisees. *Journal of Counseling Psychology*, *52*(1), 3.

James, I. A. (2015). The rightful demise of the sh* t sandwich: Providing effective feedback. *Behavioural and Cognitive Psychotherapy*, *43*(6), 759–766.

Ladany, N., & Melincoff, D. S. (1999). The nature of counselor supervisor non-disclosure. *Counselor Education and Supervision*, *38*(3), 161–176.

Milne, D. (2018). *Evidence-based CBT supervision: Principles and practice* (2nd ed.). Hoboke, NJ: Wiley.

Nelson, M. L., Barnes, K. L., Evans, A. L., & Triggiano, P. J. (2008). Working with conflict in clinical supervision: Wise supervisors' perspectives. *Journal of Counseling Psychology*, *55*(2), 172.

Richman, A. (2021). Accreditation within EMDR Europe (PowerPoint presentation). *EMDR Association UK. Consultant's Training*.

Scaife, J. (2019). *Supervision in clinical practice: a practitioner's guide* (3rd ed.). Milton Park, Abingdon, Oxon: Routledge.

Shen-Miller, D. S., Schwartz-Mette, R., Van Sickle, K. S., Jacobs, S. C., Grus, C. L., Hunter, E. A., & Forrest, L. (2015). Professional competence problems in training: A qualitative investigation of trainee perspectives. *Training and Education in Professional Psychology*, *9*(2), 161.

Sobell, L. C., Manor, H. L., Sobell, M. B., & Dum, M. (2008). Self-critiques of audiotaped therapy sessions: A motivational procedure for facilitating feedback during supervision. *Training and Education in Professional Psychology*, *2*(3), 151.

Stoltenberg, C., Bailey, K. C., Cruzan, C. B., Hart, J. T., & Ukuku, U. (2014). The integrative developmental model of supervision. In C. E. Watkins Jr, & D. Milne (Eds.), *The Wiley international handbook of clinical supervision* (pp. 576–597). Malden, MA: Wiley.

Woolliscroft, J. (2021). Accreditation applications - Good practice examples. In R. Logie (Ed.), *EMDR consultants resources book* (2nd ed.). Hove, UK: Trauma Aid UK.

Chapter 7

Integrating the Educating, Enabling, and Evaluating roles

- The Supervision Question (SQ)
- Integrating the three theoretical models: functions, modes, and levels
- Asking for feedback
- Being creative in supervision

In the previous three chapters, I have covered the three functions of supervision: *Educating, Enabling,* and *Evaluating.* I will now talk about how the roles of teacher, enabler, and evaluator need to be balanced within supervision.

The Supervision Question

In Chapter 2, I introduced the concept of the Supervision Question (SQ) and promised that we would return to it in this chapter. This is because, after considering the different functions, modes, and levels of supervision (Chapter 3) and examining each of the three functions in detail (Chapters 4, 5, and 6), it is the SQ which will help us to determine which function or mode we need to work within when our supervisee presents a particular case.

Here, I just need to remind my readers of what I have already stated in Chapter 2: Often my supervisees are irritated by my insistence on them providing an SQ. They just want to tell me about their client! But the SQ provides the focus that I need as a supervisor to really help my supervisee to get what they want out of the session. It also helps me to know when to interrupt if I think that the information they are providing is irrelevant to the SQ. Sometimes just the process of formulating the SQ means that the supervisee immediately realises where they are going wrong. Some of my supervisees object to being asked the SQ as they feel this is too constraining. One way of dealing with this is to broaden the question out to something like, "why are you bringing this particular client to supervision today."

Providing the SQ can be hard work for the therapist but formulating this question in itself can be transformative and puts the therapist already on the road to understanding where they may be going wrong even before they have

DOI: 10.4324/9781003214588-8

said any more about their client. I experienced this myself when I told my supervisor that my SQ was "how can I overcome my client's resistance?" As soon as I had asked this question, I knew where I was going wrong. A supervisee once asked, "how do I solve all of his problems?" In response to this question, we both just laughed together because, as soon as she had uttered these words, she knew how she needed to reframe her relationship with her client.

Some supervisees really do not like the restraint that the SQ imposes upon them. One of my supervisees said, "you know I don't like being asked that!" to which I responded by smiling sweetly and just saying, "yes, I know" with the implication being that I have acknowledged how she feels but will still keep asking. A few meetings later, she said, "you will be pleased to know that I have a supervision question for you this week." After a few minutes, I pointed out that she had not yet posed a question to which she replied, "wait for it! It's coming!" By using humour we have managed to move towards a point where she can start to accept that the SQ may sometimes be useful.

Sometimes the question might be something like, "just validation really." Whilst strictly speaking, this is not a question, it is clear what the supervisee is asking for in relation to this particular presentation.

How frustrating can politicians be, when they are being interviewed and they say, in order to avoid the line of enquiry, "that's not the question you should be asking." However, as supervisors, I believe that is sometimes the most helpful thing we can say in response to the SQ once we have an idea of what the relevant issues are in relation to a particular client. One of the reasons why the therapist might be stuck with a particular client is because they are asking the *wrong* SQ. This is where awareness of the functions (Educating/Enabling/Evaluating), modes (Seven-Eyes), and levels (Developmental) can be helpful. For example, the SQ might be, "have I chosen the right target for my client?", a question that lies in the mode of *Eye Two: the therapy*. However, after receiving further information from the therapist, the supervisor may realise that they have not really taken a thorough history, do not have a coherent formulation, and have rushed into doing the processing. The real question needs to be in *Eye One: the client*. Until we really understand what is happening in terms of formulation, we cannot decide on an appropriate target for processing and, indeed, such a target is likely to become obvious once we have a clear formulation.

As well as being clear about the SQ, it is important for the supervisor to ascertain whether the question has actually been answered when the discussion is completed. I have found, from my own experience, that the best way of getting feedback from the supervisee is to ask, "how does that feel now?" Notice that I am asking for feedback at an emotional level rather than at a cognitive level. This is because, until the supervisee feels differently about their client and their course of action, our interaction will not lead to any real change in relation to this particular client or to my supervisee's understanding and practice in general. Think about how this relates to EMDR therapy where we are working with an NC that has an emotional charge and we are asking, in relation to the Positive Cognition (PC), "how true do those words *feel* …?" Obviously if they are hitting themselves on the head and exclaiming, "oh I see! I get it now!" asking for feedback may be superfluous.

Integrating the three theoretical models: Functions, modes, and levels

The process of clinical supervision is a very complex one and I can imagine some readers exclaiming, "I have enough to think about during supervision without also trying to work out which function, mode or level we are in!" Once again let us look at how this corresponds to what occurs in therapy. During a session of therapy, the therapist cannot possibly be fully aware of all that is going on, holding in mind the content of what their client is saying, their formulation, plans as to what to do next, their own feelings about the client, the therapeutic relationship, and so on. Often it is not until we reflect on what has happened after the session, alone or with a colleague or supervisor, that we realise what has been occurring. Similarly, in supervision, there is so much going on that one cannot possibly be aware of everything that is relevant. However, understanding and knowing the theories behind supervision will enable the supervisor to work more effectively and also to respond sometimes instinctively; the supervisor may only fully understand what has occurred until after the session or during their own supervision of supervision.

What follows are a couple of examples of how an understanding of the functions, modes, and levels of supervision can be helpful to the supervisor.

The novice EMDR therapist

Let us start with a supervisee who has just completed their basic seven-day training. Their SQ is as follows: "Is my client ready to start EMDR processing?"

Obviously, the supervisor will need to know more about the client, the formulation, and what has been done in terms of preparation. But immediately we hear this question there are some things to think about: The therapist is clearly at *Level 1 (Dependency stage for EMDR therapists)* in terms of their development as an EMDR therapist although they may be very experienced in other modes of therapy. The question relates to what they should do with their client, so, in terms of the mode, we are working within *Eye Two (The therapy)*. And finally, which function are we in? At face value, it looks like the *Educating* function because the therapist is asking a question about what they should do. However, the subtext may be that it is really around the therapist's trepidation about starting EMDR processing, in which case this really relates to the *Enabling* function. And it may be that we have never supervised this therapist before, so there are still issues of trust and, in fact, the more relevant mode may be *Eye Five (The supervisory relationship)*.

As a supervisor in this situation, I may tell the therapist a story about when I started out as an EMDR therapist, how scary it was when I began the Desensitization phase with my first client, but how well it actually went and how delighted I was with the outcome. I would then advise the therapist that they had a good formulation, their client is adequately prepared and would exclaim, "crack on!" So, I would be presenting myself as a coping model in order to address the therapist's fears before giving them the encouragement to start processing.

The aspiring EMDR consultant

The second vignette relates to a therapist who trained in EMDR seven years ago and has been an accredited Practitioner for four years. They do not wish to discuss a particular client but, instead, to ask you why you have not yet agreed to recommend them for accreditation as an EMDR Consultant.

The therapist presents as having a high opinion of themselves and their therapeutic skills. When they do bring a client to supervision, it is usually in order to demonstrate how skilled they are as a therapist rather than to ask for help with a particular point of stuckness. They have attended the Consultant's Training and the report from this training outlined a number of issues that they needed to work on, particularly an inadequate grasp of the Standard Protocol and a tendency, in supervision, to patronise the supervisee and give advice which does not bear any relation to the SQ. The therapist denies that these are issues that need to be addressed and says that the tutor on the Consultants Training "had it in for me."

In terms of their level of development, one would expect this therapist to be at *Level 3 (Conditional dependency)* but they may, in fact, still be at the previous stage of *Level 2 (Dependency-autonomy)*. At this level, the supervisee fluctuates between feeling overconfident and feeling overwhelmed. In this particular example, it appears that the therapist has developed narcissistic overconfidence as a coping strategy to deal with occasions when, in fact, they feel overwhelmed. In terms of the function, we are clearly looking at the *Evaluating* realm because the issue is whether the supervisor will agree to sign their accreditation form. In terms of the mode, we appear to be in *Eye Five (The supervisory relationship)*. The quality of the supervisory relationship, like the quality of the therapeutic relationship, is highly dependent on trust and respect. We may also be dealing with the therapist's own issues which relate to previous unresolved events in terms of their education or earlier family relationships, in other words, *Eye Four (The therapist's "stuff")*. But the supervisor's own issues may also be affecting what is happening here (*Eye Six. The supervisor's "stuff"*).

In such a situation the supervisor's first task is, perhaps, to do some work on themselves in order that they do not become too emotionally involved in what is going on. They need to accept, perhaps, that they cannot be held in high regard by all their supervisees. Discussing it with their own supervisor may assist with this. Secondly, the supervisor may need to give the therapist some very concrete and specific feedback about what they still need to work on and how this might be achieved. This needs to be done with acceptance of the strong possibility that this feedback may be rejected and the therapist may leave them and seek another supervisor. The specific feedback may consist of a written list of bullet points, for example, regarding how to brush up on the Standard Protocol and critically reflect on their own videos of supervision sessions regarding the supervisory relationship. Again, telling a story about a time when the supervisor, themselves, had to deal with negative feedback and respond to it in an appropriate way might also help to ensure that the therapist actually hears what the supervisor is saying.

Asking for feedback

In order to be an effective supervisor, it is my belief that it is important to briefly ask for the supervisee's feedback after the presentation of each case or supervisory dilemma. As I described in the section above regarding the SQ, the feedback should always relate to the original SQ to find out, at least, whether it has been answered. I will ask questions such as, "was that helpful?" or, more significantly, "how does that feel now?"

Why do I ask my supervisee how they feel rather than whether they understand things differently? Let us refer back again to what occurs in EMDR therapy. The Negative Cognition and Positive Cognition in EMDR both contain an emotional element as well as being just cognitions. When reprocessing occurs during therapy, the cognitive shift encapsulates an emotional shift. For example, changing from "I am worthless" to "I am OK as I am" includes a significant emotional shift as well as a change in cognitive appraisal. If we translate that into what may occur in a supervision session, our supervisee may shift from "I don't know where I am going with this client and I'm feeling useless" to "aha! I know what to do now. Now I am looking forward to their next therapy session." So that is why I ask my supervisee how they feel. Only if there has been an emotional shift will the supervisee have learnt from this piece of supervision and, more crucially be able to generalise it to other clients in the future.

Sometimes I hardly need to ask the feedback question as it is obvious from my supervisee's demeanour that some shift has occurred or they have already said, "that was really helpful." At other times their nonverbal language may be enough to tell that I have been unable to help them as yet. If they are frowning or appearing frustrated with my response to their SQ I am alerted to the fact that we are not there yet. Once again, using EMDR therapy as an analogy, I may need to identify the blocking belief that is preventing my supervisee from "getting it."

There have been occasions when I have to confess to my supervisee that I don't have a solution to their SQ. On every such occasion, when my request for feedback was, "I am sorry, I don't think I've been of much help on this one," the reply has invariably been along the lines of, "no, actually it has been very helpful to know that Robin doesn't have the answer either which make me feel a whole lot better!" Sometimes what we are teaching our supervisees in such cases is the importance of living with uncertainty in the therapy room.

However, it should be accepted that cultural issues may be at play here. For example, when supervising a group of supervisees from Cambodia, Laos, Vietnam, and China, Masuma Rahim was expected to be their ultimate authority. When she asked how she could improve her supervision, the supervisees were offended and she was scolded for asking because she was expected to know how to supervise them (Yabusaki, 2010).

Being creative in supervision

The more creative one can be as a supervisor, the more rewarding the supervisory experience is likely to be for both parties. When are we most creative during EMDR therapy? Well, in my view, it is when we are using interweaves. So, it may be helpful to think of our feedback to supervisees as a kind of interweave. And, talking of interweaves, a supervisee, already very experienced in CBT, said that he had got stuck during an EMDR session and just felt like he wanted to revert to CBT. I felt stuck myself at this moment and asked, more out of curiosity than anything else, what he would have done if he had reverted to CBT. "Aha! I see what I need to do now!" he exclaimed. I had no idea what I had said or done to help him until he explained that he realised that he needed to use an interweave and that an interweave is "just a little bit of CBT."

There follows some of my own ideas about doing supervision in a more creative way.

Borders and Brown (2005) refer to "thinking aloud" as a way of responding to supervisee's questions. To be honest, I sometimes use this approach when I am unsure about how to respond to my supervisee's question. I will say, "I'm just going to think aloud now, so what I say may not make much sense at first." In my experience, what then happens is that the supervisee joins in with my musings and somehow, together, we reach a satisfactory answer to their SQ. To quote Joyce Scaife, this is the process of being with someone "who is happy to wade with me in the murky swamp." Scaife (2019, p. 4).

As already mentioned in Chapter 4, I have a particular interest in the storytelling approach in EMDR therapy (Logie et al., 2020) and it will therefore come as no surprise that I tell stories in supervision too. Rather than answer the question directly I will tell a story, usually about one of my own clients, in order to illustrate the point that I wish to make. More often than not, I do not need to spell out what the message is that the story conveys, and my supervisee is already nodding in realisation of how they may approach things differently. I would encourage you to try the same: Be open to what you are being reminded of as your supervisee talks to you. Does it resonate with something that has happened in your own work or in your life generally? Do you think it would be helpful for your supervisee to hear the story? Sometimes I am unsure, and I preface the story with, "this has reminded me of something that happened to me. I'm not sure if it will be helpful to you if I share it, but let's find out!"

Conclusion

The three functions of Educating, Enabling, and Evaluating will never occur separately as discrete activities. As supervisors, we need to accept that more than one of these may be relevant at any particular moment. We also need to be cognisant as to which of the Seven Eyes is in focus. Also, the supervisee's level of development may be relevant to what is being discussed in supervision.

As I have said, the reflection often can only come after the session. However, at an online Consultants Day in the UK, I did ask the participants to actually supervise each other on a case during the workshop directly after I had outlined the theory. I asked them to be aware of what was happening in these brief sessions. Some of the feedback was that the exercise had helped them to think about supervision in a different way and one participant posted in the chat facility, "we are always learning, the process is complex and multi-layered, and some treasure to be had whichever level is coming up/being explored."

Borders, L. D., & Brown, L. L. (2005). *The new handbook of counseling supervision.* New York, NY: Routledge

Logie, R., Bowers, M., Dent, A., Elliot, J., O'Connor, M., & Russell, A. (2020). *Using stories in EMDR. A guide to the storytelling (narrative) approach in EMDR therapy.* Brighton, UK: Trauma Aid UK.

Scaife, J. (2019). *Supervision in clinical practice: A practitioner's guide* (3rd ed.). Milton Park, Abingdon, Oxon: Routledge.

Yabusaki, A. S. (2010). Clinical supervision: Dialogues on diversity. *Training and Education in Professional Psychology, 4*(1), 55.

Chapter 8

Challenges in supervision

- Diversity
- Supervisee "resistance"
- Rupture and repair
- Getting the level right
- Unsatisfactory performance

I am speculating that some people, when picking up this book for the first time, will go straight to this section before reading any other part of the book in their quest to find an answer to a difficulty that they are having with a particular supervisee. I understand that this may be tempting, but without understanding the theory and reading much of what has gone before, they may not realise that the answers to their questions will be contained throughout the book. In fact, there are no easy answers. In some ways, this book will hopefully enable EMDR Consultants to take a step back and understand better what is happening in supervision generally which will mean that they will then intuitively find the answers themselves to some of the trickier problems. Once again, there is a parallel here with what actually happens during EMDR processing: We do not give answers to our clients' dilemmas but instead we put them in a place where the answers will become apparent and, much more powerfully, they will find the answers themselves.

I guess there will be other individuals who might pick up this book and be thinking, "why so complicated? Isn't EMDR supervision just a matter of teaching them how to do EMDR and making sure that they get it right?" Well, yes, for a minority of supervisees, this may be all that they need. Compare this to EMDR therapy itself: Some EMDR therapy sessions can be very straightforward. (My son-in-law, a photographer with a degree in engineering, who provided technical support for my online trainings, on observing me doing a demonstration of EMDR remarked, "it looks pretty simple really. You just wave your hand, ask them 'what do you get now' and then then say 'go with that'"!) In some EMDR therapy sessions we may require no interweaves and the SUD may quickly go to 0 and the VOC to 7. But how often does that actually happen in real life? It is more normal to

DOI: 10.4324/9781003214588-9

encounter blocking beliefs, feeder memories, and other obstacles along the way. Similarly, in EMDR supervision, the supervisee's ability to understand and effectively use the Standard Protocol may be blocked by their difficulty in letting go of their well-learned previous therapeutic modalities, their fear of their client's abreactions, their fear of being judged by their supervisor, and so on. Therefore, in order just to enable the therapist to effectively use EMDR, a complex understanding of the process of supervision may be required.

The two vignettes that I outlined in the previous chapter entitled "Integrating the three theoretical models: functions, modes, and levels," illustrate two contrasting situations in which there is a lack of a collaborative relationship in the supervision room. In the first vignette ("Is my client ready to start EMDR processing?"), the supervisee is expressing that they feel incompetent, and they may become over-reliant on always checking things out with their supervisor when, in fact, they know exactly what to do. By complete contrast, the second vignette is about a supervisee who has developed a narcissistic way of coping with their sense of incompetence. In contrasting ways, both individuals are unlikely to learn or develop much if they become stuck in these roles and it is the supervisor's role to help to free them. In those two vignettes, I have suggested some possible ways in which the supervisor could transform the supervisory relationship into one that will work better for the supervisee.

Diversity

I have attempted, in this book, to be mindful of issues of diversity wherever it arises. However, I believe that it is useful to spend some time focusing on this issue specifically in this chapter relating to Challenges in Supervision.

Firstly, this has been one of the hardest parts of this book to write. Sharing my own difficulties with my readers will, I believe, be helpful in learning and understanding some of the considerations that diversity can pose.

My problem with diversity seems to be that have what I call a "diversity blind spot" and have tended to react to questions of diversity by thinking "I don't know what the issue is. I just treat everyone the same. Isn't that enough?" Is this ringing any bells with some of my readers? I am a white middle-class man brought up in a comfortable intact family. There was discrimination and related trauma in a previous generation as my mother was a Jewish refugee fleeing from Nazi Germany as a 19-year-old. But I was protected from that. My father was not Jewish, and I was brought up with no religion. In fact, rather than feeling like a member of a persecuted group, I have become aware that my Jewish origins may have engendered in me a sense of superiority with the Jewish belief that we are God's "chosen people" (Deuteronomy 7:6).

It has only been the process of writing this book which has forced me into starting to think about this. I have been particularly helped by a colleague explaining to me, over a pint in the pub after an EMDR training, about "white privilege" or, more generally "social privilege." This refers to any advantage based on education, social class, caste, age, height, weight, nationality, geographic location, disability, ethnic or racial category, gender, gender identity, neurology, sexual orientation, physical attractiveness, religion, or other differentiating factors (Black & Stone, 2005). For more reading on this, I would recommend the excellent book, *White Privilege Unmasked* by Judy Ryde (Ryde, 2019).

Like many others, I have been unaware of the advantages that have been conferred upon me by my background. The privilege is often unconscious, and this lack of awareness obviously makes it all the more pernicious (McIntosh, 2019).

So how might this be relevant to EMDR supervision? Ryde (2019) points out that it is unusual …

> … for the question in supervision to be "how do you think your being white impacts on this situation?" It is more usual to ask "how do you think this person feels about being black in this situation?" The first question puts the focus on the white person and how their whiteness influences the dynamic. By looking at the issues in this way we can start to address some of the responsibility that white people have within a racial context. It makes the issue theirs as much as others and implicitly brings the unequal power dynamic to the fore. When we ask a black person how they feel, or wonder how the black client feels, there is an implicit assumption that they are "different" within a "normal" context. This can subtly emphasize and reinforce the dynamic of the white person being the "normal" one and therefore the most powerful.
>
> (Ryde, 2019)

So, what are the specific issues relating to diversity that we should be aware of as EMDR supervisors? Firstly, I believe that the main issue relates to the power relationship in supervision that results from the Evaluating component of EMDR supervision where the supervisor acts as gatekeeper regarding the supervisee's readiness to become an accredited Practitioner or Consultant. Where the diversity of the supervisee (their gender, race, sexual orientation, and so on) causes an additional power imbalance in the supervisory relationship, it is important for both supervisor and supervisee to be aware of what the potential impact might be.

Secondly, it should be noted that some therapists will not be receiving any supervision other than for EMDR. Also, they may be presenting cases to their EMDR supervisor where issues of diversity may arise in relation to the client or in the supervisory relationship. Whilst such issues may not relate directly to the technicalities of EMDR, they may be getting in the way of the therapy (the therapeutic relationship – "Eye 3" of the Seven-Eyed model) or the supervisory relationship ("Eye 5"). In that case, they need to be addressed.

To what extent should supervisors work only with supervisees and clients who are from a similar cultural background? As well as the practical impossibility of always doing so, it is probably more important that supervisors cultivate a willingness and curiosity about looking at such issues between themselves and their supervisees. Scaife (2019) describes the "continuous effort and imagination" (p. 183) that is required in order to address issues of difference.

We must also be aware that we should never make assumptions and second-guess what we might think the issues are likely to be. As one of my colleagues said, "as a person of Indian descent and Caribbean birth, I might think that I 'know' where my Trinidadian client is coming from while unwittingly turning a blind eye to the fact that she is of a different generation, of a different social class and religion and grew up in the sheltered confines of an elite secondary school in another country." Similarly, as someone with a Jewish mother, meaning that I am technically Jewish, you would think that I might have felt some connection to a client I saw some years ago, who was an Orthodox Jew. Not only did I feel a massive cultural gulf between us, I also felt it important not to disclose my heritage as he might assume that I had extraordinary knowledge and understanding of his situation *vis a vis* his religious identity, before discovering that I was not *properly* Jewish!

So, what can we actually do as supervisors to address these issues? The following is based on list of considerations provided by Scaife (2019):

Noticing how you feel

Firstly, notice feelings of discomfort and embarrassment in relation to the experience of difference between you and your supervisee and give full attention to them. An example of this might be a feeling of uncertainty as to whether to mention the race of your supervisee when you think it might be a relevant issue in relation to the client being discussed and, if so, what word to use (e.g. "black," "brown," "person of colour").

Educating yourself and your supervisee

If you do not know what you believe that you need to know about your supervisee's gender, culture, sexual orientation, disability, and so, then ASK them! Similarly, suggest to your supervisees that they do the same with their clients. Point out to them that they should never make assumptions about their client's values and beliefs based upon their culture. It may be necessary to encourage your supervisee to find out how their service is monitoring referrals by gender, ethnicity, disability, age, and so on. Or what services exist for specific groups.

Explore the power dynamics

Discuss with your supervisee what might be significant about the differences between you and them and, or the supervisee and their client. All pairings will have something particular to say about privilege, for example, a black, unemployed male client with a therapist who is

- a white female
- or a black, gay male
- or a physically disabled, straight male

And then add in the characteristics of the supervisor and, perhaps, what fantasies the supervisee might have about how the supervisor perceives what they are telling them about their client in supervision.

And, finally, it is important to accept that looking at issues of diversity is hard for all of us. It is important to recognise for ourselves and acknowledge to our supervisees that we should try but we may never actually get it completely right.

Supervisee "resistance"

Bernard and Goodyear (2019) refer to "supervisee resistance" and compare it with client "resistance" in therapy. But, as in therapy, to frame any supervisee behaviour as "resistance" risks blaming the supervisee for what could be a healthy and adaptive response to perceived threat (Abernethy & Cook, 2011). Shohet (2012) reframes resistance as "feedback on something that has not yet been understood" (p. 260). Amongst other factors, Shohet describes resistance as one way in which supervisees will protect themselves against feelings of vulnerability. In practical terms, he summarises the following approaches to reducing the possibility that resistance will occur in supervision:

- Clear contracting to explain the purpose of supervision, the way of working, and sharing expectations.
- Sharing positive experiences of supervision and learning
- When noticing resistance, the supervisor being willing to check themselves out to see if they have missed something rather than blame the supervisee
- Eliciting and making explicit core beliefs
- Reframing – seeing the commitment behind the complaint
- Noticing competing commitments and making them explicit
- Recognising parallel process whereby the supervisee begins to present in the same way as their patient has presented to them. In other words, recognising that the resistance can go from patient, to supervisee, to supervisor

- Naming the potential for sabotage right at the beginning
(Shohet, 2012, p. 281)

Much of what occurs in supervisee resistance relates to shame (Kearns, 2018). As EMDR therapists we are all too well aware of shame-related Negative Cognitions (NCs) such as "I am not good enough" and such cognitions and their accompanying emotions will often enter the supervision room. Supervision is likely to elicit shame due to its Evaluating component. In addition, it involves the fear of being exposed in the context of a bond where the supervisee values the opinion of the supervisor (Bernard & Goodyear, 2019). Supervisees may respond to their own feelings of shame either passively through withdrawal and avoidance or aggressively by criticising their supervisor or themselves.

Rupture and repair

The longest supervisory relationship that I have experienced has been with my wife, Jane Logie, since training together as clinical psychologists and meeting for peer supervision in 1982. The romantic relationship actually came later! Now retired from her career as a clinical child psychologist, I still turn to Jane on occasions for help with children with whom I am working who have early attachment-related trauma, which Jane had specialised in. During the early stages of writing this book an uncharacteristic rupture occurred in our supervisory relationship and we agreed to independently write an account of what occurred:

Robin's experience

I asked Jane for some supervision regarding Ben today. I thought it was just a straightforward question about a resource she might be able to recommend regarding ways to help him to self-regulate.

My SQ was, "can you recommend any resources (books or programmes) for parents to help a child learn ways of self-regulating?" I was instantly disappointed by her response as she started to do a sort of lecture about how children learn to self-regulate and how they miss out on this stage in their early development if they have early attachment-related trauma. "Yeah, yeah", I thought. "I know all that, but how can we actually teach Ben to learn to self-regulate." I may have, sort of, expressed some of this out loud! Jane was starting to look a bit tense and seemed to be just repeating herself and saying the same thing in more detail. So, I asked, what the parents should actually do. I still felt we were on different wavelengths, so I asked her if she could give me an example. She declined to do this so I gave her an example of a situation which might occur when Ben loses his temper. Jane told me that it wasn't the time to be teaching him self-regulation and that he needs to learn it when he is calmer and hasn't lost the plot. "But", I said, "what do we actually do or say to Ben when he is calmer?" "Well, usually when I explain this to the parents, they understand what I am talking about and we come up with an idea together." I still didn't understand what she was telling me so, off the top of my head, I came up with the following scenario:

So, for example, you might say, "Ben? Are you listening to me? Yes? Good. We are going to play a game of xxx in a few minutes, but I need to finish loading the dishwasher first. I want you to try really hard and stay calm and wait for me while I load the dishwasher. If you are still calm when I've finished, we will play the game." Then just leave him to his own devices whilst you load the dishwasher. If he has been able to stay calm, say, "wow, Ben, that's amazing! You managed to stay calm. I'm really pleased with you. Now, let's play that game."

"Yes", said Jane, "I think you are getting it now."

Aaagh! So why didn't she tell me that in the first place? Well, maybe I had to work it out for myself.

Jane's experience

Robin asked me for some supervision about Ben and his family. He said it was just a question and may only take a minute or so or it may develop into a longer discussion.

Robin told me that Ben's parents are asking how they can help Ben learn to regulate his emotions rather than going from 0–60 when he is feeling angry. Ben does not want to be like this – how can they help him? Do I know of a book or manual?

I had a sinking, overwhelmed feeling that this is impossible for Ben to achieve and thought, 'where are we going to start with it?' I attempted some kind of answer about the process of learning that he has missed out on with examples. Robin stated that he didn't understand. I continued and the same happened again.

I then felt panicky – that I didn't know what I was talking about. I recovered and rather than giving suggestions, asked Robin what he thought Ben needed to learn in order to have more success at being able to regulate his emotions. It then felt that we started working together on some joined up understanding and ideas about providing regular re-learning experiences.

Thinking about it afterwards our supervision seemed to reflect the experience that many adoptive parents have of thinking that there are ways of fixing these children if only they knew how – and other people know and is being kept from them – like conception and having their own baby kept from them.

The rupture started to occur immediately when Jane recognised that the way in which my SQ was framed was actually getting in the way of me helping my client. She tried to re-frame the dilemma, but I remained stuck in my way of thinking and Jane therefore started to feel helpless. At this point, we both needed to take a step back and look at a new way of going forward which would work. Although we both needed to do this it was Jane's primary responsibility, as supervisor, to make the first move. When she asked "what Ben needed to learn in order to have more success at being able to regulate his emotions" she was helping me to reframe the problem, rather like a cognitive interweave in EMDR therapy. At this point the repair began to occur and the supervisory relationship began to run more smoothly, both our levels of arousal came down to the point where we could subsequently reflect on what had happened between us and we could happily go away and write up what we had experienced.

"Moments of resistance or rupture occur in all authentic and meaningful relationships" (Corrie & Lane, 2015, p. 129). In fact, Lesser (1983) suggests that we should be wary of a supervisory relationship that appears too comfortable.

Safran et al. (2008) discuss rupture and repair in supervision with reference to how this occurs in therapy. They state that the rupture will start when the client sees the action of the therapist as confirming their own expectations about relationships. The client will react by confronting the therapist or by becoming withdrawn. The therapist will then react either defensively or angrily which will confirm the client's expectations. Firstly, the therapist needs to notice the rupture and then stand back from it in order to discuss it with their client.

Watkins (2021) describes two kinds of rupture in the supervisory relationship. Firstly, "confrontational" ruptures involve the supervisee criticising some aspect of the supervision. Secondly, "withdrawal" rupture "involve supervisees disengaging or pulling back from supervision or being overly appeasing" (p. 4). Watkins says that this second form of rupture is actually more common because of supervision's power-disproportionate nature. Supervisees may generally become less involved, asking fewer questions and limiting engagement with the supervisor. Conversely, they may become more compliant and deferential. Because withdrawal ruptures are more indirect, by definition, they can be more difficult to identify and may take a period of time to detect.

Rupture will sometimes occur in the context of issues regarding diversity or cultural differences. This issue was examined in a study by Lubbers (2013) in which supervisors were reported to have made insulting, racist and homophobic comments such as, "Well, those beliefs are supernatural and not based at all in science, so you probably should not discuss religion with your clients because your beliefs will harm your clinical work" (p. 79).

Grant et al. (2012) interviewed 16 experienced supervisors. This is a summary of the ways in which they managed ruptures in the supervisory relationship:

- Name the difficulty
  - Be explicit about the issue and bring it out into the open
- Validate and normalise
  - Explain that what the supervisee is experiencing is understandable and normal

- Attune to the supervisee's needs
  - Accept that the supervisee is needing something from the supervision, even if you believe they should not need to!
- Support
  - Provide support in difficult situations such as a suicidal client
- Anticipate
  - Be aware of what potential difficulties may arise in the supervisory relationship before they happen
- Explore parallel process
  - Draw parallels between what is happening in supervision and what may be occurring in the therapeutic relationship
- Acknowledge mistakes
  - Be open about the things that you have got wrong in the supervisory relationship
- Modelling
  - Actually enact in the supervision what the supervisee needs to do. For example, disclosing your own mistakes may help the supervisee to be more open about theirs.
- Facilitate reflectively
  - Reflect openly about what is happening in the supervisory relationship
- Remain mindful and monitor
  - Be aware of one's own feeling during supervision and how one is feeling towards the supervisee
- Remain patient and transparent
  - Managing supervisees' wariness, defensiveness, incompatible pace, and resistance by noticing them being open about what you are seeing
- Process countertransference
  - Being aware of and dealing with whatever is coming up for you during supervision
- Seek supervision on supervision
  - Discussing issues with one's own supervisor
- Case conceptualise
  - Help the supervisee to understand what is happening by sharing discussion about case conceptualisation

Finally, although both parties need to engage in any resolution of the rupture, rather like the parent being the person who should take the first step in a parent/child rupture, it should always be the supervisor who takes the first step, if necessary, in resolving a rupture in a supervisory relationship.

Watkins (2021) quotes Safran et al. (2019) who suggest a number of approaches that supervisors can take in order to repair ruptures: The supervisor:

- changes tasks or goals
- provides a rationale for supervision
- invites the supervisee to discuss thoughts or feelings with respect to the supervisor or some aspect of supervision
- acknowledges their contribution to the rupture
- discloses their internal experience of the supervisee-supervisor interaction
- responds by validating the supervisee's defensive posture
- responds by redirecting or refocusing the supervisee

"The reality, however, is that rupture repair can be messy, difficult, and far from simple ... Thus, it would seem a given that a back-and-forth process across steps over time – where sometimes we have to take steps backward and reassess in order to move forward – can be necessary for true repair to take hold" (Watkins, 2021, p. 9). And the most difficult part of this, according to Watkins, is for the supervisor to be "humble" (Schein & Schein, 2021).

Finally let me tell you how I would approach two different kinds of ruptures within the supervisory relationship myself. Both these stories are fictitious although they include elements of issues that have arisen with my own supervisees or with those to whom I have provided metasupervision.

Clare and Charles

Clare, the supervisee, has recently completed her basic EMDR training and has only met her supervisor, Charles, on three sessions so far. Clare is very competent and has a good grasp of the EMDR protocol but is also very anxious about working with this new model and, particularly, about the potential unpredictability of her clients' responses to EMDR processing. When she raises her anxiety with Charles, he replies with comments such as, "well, you are clearly an excellent therapist and you know the protocol so well that I don't see why you need to be so worried!" Charles presents himself as an experienced and skilled EMDR therapist who has never made any mistakes. He just hopes that by modelling himself in this way and telling Clare how good she is, she will gradually absorb some of his confidence and be able to start using EMDR with her clients. However, this approach causes Clare to feel increasingly de-skilled and she copes by becoming withdrawn in supervision, telling Charles that everything is going fine, and she has nothing much to bring to supervision.

Things come to a head when Clare mentions that she is seeking a new supervisor. At this point Charles realises for the first time that there has been a rupture in the supervisory relationship and asks Clare to describe how she feels during supervision. She tells Charles that she feels very anxious during supervision and that this is becoming worse rather than better over time. She feels that Charles believes that she is pathetic and has a poor opinion of her. Charles reacts by saying that he is very surprised by this. He shares with Clare the fact that he felt very uncertain when he started doing EMDR himself but coped with this by pretending to his own supervisor that he was doing fine due to his feelings of shame at the time. Clare was equally surprised to hear this as she assumed that Charles has been born super-confident. After this, Clare felt more able to show her vulnerability during supervision and Charles also changed by sharing more of his own experiences and what he had learned from when things had gone wrong.

Tracey and Rakhee

Rakhee has just been accredited as an EMDR Consultant and has not yet put anyone forward for accreditation. She is approached by Tracey whose last supervisor said she was not yet ready for accreditation. Tracey believes she is a competent EMDR therapist and approaches Rakhee because she believes she might be a "soft touch" and might be persuaded to put her forward for accreditation. Rakhee is aware of the importance of asking the SQ but, every time she does so, Tracey rolls her eyes and says, "do I *have* to?" Rakhee tentatively asks Tracey if she can provide a video of her work, but Tracey provides a string of excuses such as the client not giving consent or technical problems. Rakhee tries to cope with Tracey by being empathic and understanding. But as she does so, Tracey becomes increasingly challenging and Rakhee feels increasingly out of control during supervision sessions.

Eventually Rakhee takes this to her own supervisor to discuss. Much to her surprise, her supervisor tells her that her supervisee currently has little respect for her and, if she sets firm limits and takes more control of the supervision sessions, Tracey will feel safer and be able to make more use of the sessions. At the next supervision session Rakhee suggests that they pause to discuss the supervisory relationship and asks Tracey what she actually hopes to achieve from her supervision sessions. After this Tracey starts to come to supervision with a different attitude in which she wants to actually learn and develop as an EMDR therapist.

Getting the level right

Rakhee might have benefitted from reading the research by Ögren, Boalt Boëthius, and Olsson (2008) which indicates that being "nice" and "accepting" is not necessarily appreciated by supervisees. Supervisors were appreciated more if they were "straightforward, expressed empathy, and held an autonomous position that conveyed their care about how things turned out for their students and their clients" (Ögren & Boalt Boëthius, 2014, pp. 354–355). They added that being a "containing authority" was appreciated by supervisees. I have already quoted Fleming et al. (2007) who warn that supervision can become "devoid of critical reflection, mutate into backslapping and become part of what has been called the 'tyranny of niceness'" (p. 22). A study by Rieck et al. (2015) showed that client outcome was better when low supervisor agreeableness was present.

However, Ogren and Boalt Boëthius (2014) also point out that becoming too authoritarian and proclaiming that only they know the "absolute truth" was also unhelpful to supervisees. In fact, it is all a matter of getting the level right for each particular supervisee. Whilst too much anxiety can affect what supervisees can notice and encode (Dombeck & Brody, 1995), just the right amount of anxiety in the supervision room will be optimal for effective supervision. As an undergraduate, I recall learning about the Yerkes and Dodson (1908) famous hypothesis that both too little or too much arousal will reduce the ability to perform a task. Again, we are reminded here of the "window of tolerance" concept we use in EMDR processing (Siegel, 1999). I have attempted to explain this in the diagram below. I hope this is useful although I accept that the lowest area which I have named "too laid-back to learn" does not quite equate with hypo-arousal.

Unsatisfactory performance

There will always be situations when no amount of discussion about the supervisory relationship or attempts by the supervisor to address the issues will be sufficient. Sometimes the supervisor will be faced with a decision about how to manage their supervisee's unsatisfactory performance as an EMDR therapist. Forrest et al. (1999) introduced three main categories of unsatisfactory performance which are summarised by Beinart and Clohessy (2017) as follows:

- Incompetence
- Unethical practice
- Lack of professional competence or impairment

Incompetence is the one we are most often likely to come across and the easiest to deal with. Although painful for supervisees to hear, to highlight the areas in which competence has not been achieved can be helpful in identifying where further learning needs to happen. This was largely covered in the previous chapter regarding the Evaluating function of supervision.

Unethical practice refers to the infringement of professional codes of ethics or codes of conduct such as entering into a sexual relationship with a

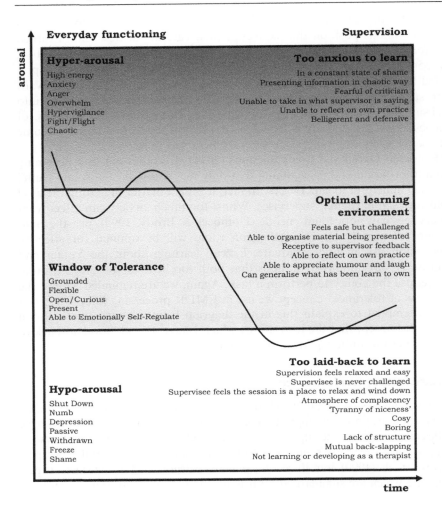

Figure 8.1 The "Window of Tolerance" in EMDR supervision.

client. As EMDR Consultants we do not usually have managerial responsibility for our supervisees and it would, in any event, be for the accrediting body of their core profession to deal with such issues. However, it will be our ethical duty to report concerns that we may have regarding unethical practice to the supervisee's manager or professional body.

Lack of professional competence or impairment differs from incompetence in that it refers to diminished functioning due to extreme personal distress and due to such things as alcohol or substance misuse. However Falender and Shafranske (2007) suggest that the use of the word "impairment" is unsuitable as it has a specific legal definition with relation to disability.

Gilfoyle (2008) proposes ten best practice guidelines for managing poor practice:

- provide written standards or competencies against which performance will be measured (usually provided by the training or regulatory body)
- have written policies of procedures to deal with competency problems
- follow procedures and document meetings
- apply standards fairly and ethically, and follow due process
- establish internal review processes and respect confidentiality as far as possible
- stay focused on problems in relation to training or professional goals
- design remediation plans in line with programme or professional criteria and goals
- consider safety for all involved
- keep a written record of all interactions and decisions
- do not delay in addressing problems

Conclusion

Hopefully this chapter will have provided some help in relation to some very tricky areas in EMDR supervision. But unfortunately, it will have provided no easy answers to some very thorny dilemmas about how to manage things when they go wrong in supervision. As I write this, I am thinking about the feeling I have during supervision when I believe that I have been of little help to my supervisee. I am actually wondering what Jane might say if I brought this to supervision with her. She would probably say, as she has done so many times before, "Robin, you need to accept that not every problem is solvable and sometimes we just have to stay with it and share the discomfort." In other words, "just notice"!

Abernethy, C., & Cook, K. (2011). Resistance or disconnection? A relational-cultural approach to supervisee anxiety and nondisclosure. *Journal of Creativity in Mental Health*, 6(1), 2–14.

Beinart, H., & Clohessy, S. (2017). *Effective supervisory relationships. Best evidence and practice.* Chichester, UK: Wiley.

Bernard, J. M., & Goodyear, R. K. (2019). *Fundimentals of clinical supervision* (6th ed.). New York, NY: Pearson.

Black, L. L., & Stone, D. (2005). Expanding the definition of privilege: The concept of social privilege. *Journal of Multicultural Counseling and Development*, 33(4), 243–255.

Corrie, S., & Lane, D. (2015). *CBT supervision.* London: Sage.

Dombeck, M.-T., & Brody, S. L. (1995). Clinical supervision: A three-way mirror. *Archives of Psychiatric Nursing, 9*(1), 3–10.

Falender, C. A., & Shafranske, E. P. (2007). Competence in competency-based supervision practice: Construct and application. *Professional Psychology: Research and Practice, 38*(3), 232.

Fleming, I., Gone, R., Diver, A., & Fowler, B. (2007). Risk supervision in Rochdale. *Clinical Psychology Forum, 176,* 22–25.

Forrest, L., Elman, N., Gizara, S., & Vacha-Haase, T. (1999). Trainee impairment: A review of identification, remediation, dismissal, and legal issues. *The Counseling Psychologist, 27*(5), 627–686.

Gilfoyle, N. (2008). The legal exosystem: Risk management in addressing student competence problems in professional psychology training. *Training and Education in Professional Psychology, 2*(4), 202.

Grant, J., Schofield, M. J., & Crawford, S. (2012). Managing difficulties in supervision: Supervisors' perspectives. *Journal of Counseling Psychology, 59*(4), 528.

Kearns, A. (2018). *The seven deadly sins?: Issues in clinical practice and supervision for humanistic and integrative practitioners.* New York, NY: Routledge.

Lesser, R. M. (1983). Supervision: Illusions, anxieties, and questions. *Contemporary Psychoanalysis, 19,* 120–129.

Lubbers, L. (2013). *Supervisees' experiences of ruptures in multicultural supervision: A qualitative study.* (PhD thesis), Milwaukee, WI: Marquette University.

McIntosh, P. (2019). White privilege: Unpacking the invisible knapsack (1989). In P. McIntosh (Ed.), *On privilege, fraudulence, and teaching as learning.* New York: Routledge.

Ogren, M., & Boalt Boëthius, S. (2014). Developing understanding in clinical supervision. In C. E. Watkins Jr & D. Milne (Eds.), *Wiley international handbook of clinical supervision* (pp. 342–363). Chichester, W. Sussex: Wiley.

Ögren, M.-L., Boalt Boëthius, S., & Olsson, U. (2008). Organizational structure and framework: A case study of Swedish training programs in psychotherapy. *Organizational and Social Dynamics, 8*(22), 256–278.

Rieck, T., Callahan, J. L., & Watkins Jr, C. E. (2015). Clinical supervision: An exploration of possible mechanisms of action. *Training and Education in Professional Psychology, 9*(2), 187.

Ryde, J. (2019). *White privilege unmasked: How to be part of the solution.* London: Jessica Kingsley Publishers.

Safran, J. D., Muran, J. C., Stevens, C., & Rothman, M. (2008). A relational approach to supervision: Addressing ruptures in the alliance. In C. A. Falender & E. P. Shafranske (Eds.), *Casebook for clinical supervision: A competency-based approach.* (pp. 137–157).

Safran, J. D., Muran, J. C., & Eubanks-Carter, C. (2019). Repairing alliance ruptures. In J. C. Norcross & M. J. Lambert (Eds.), *Psychotherapy relationships that work: Evidence-based therapist contributions* (pp. 549–579). Oxford University Press.

Scaife, J. (2019). *Supervision in clinical practice: a practitioner's guide* (3rd ed.). Milton Park, Abingdon, Oxon: Routledge.

Schein, E. H., & Schein, P. A. (2021). *Humble inquiry: The gentle art of asking instead of telling.* Oakland, CA: Berrett-Koehler Publishers.

Shohet, R. (2012). Listening to resistance. In D. Owen, & R. Shohet (Eds.), *Clinical supervision in the medical profession.* Maidenhead, UK: Open University Press.

Siegel, D. J. (1999). *The developing mind.* New York: Guilford.

Watkins, C. E. (2021). Rupture and rupture repair in clinical supervision: Some thoughts and steps along the way. *The Clinical Supervisor, 40*(2), 321–344.

Yerkes, R., & Dodson, J. (1908). The relation of strength of stimulus to rapidity of habit-formation. *Journal of Comparative Neurology and Psychology, 18*(5), 459–482.

Chapter 9

Group supervision

- Why group supervision?
- Types of groups
- How many in the group?
- Homogeneous versus heterogeneous
- The group context
- Organisation and structuring of groups
- Protocol for EMDR Group Supervision
- Brushing up on the protocol
- EMDR accreditation
- Group dynamics

In my experience, providing EMDR supervision in groups can be both rewarding for the supervisor and enriching for the supervisees. Much of the EMDR supervision that is taking place occurs in groups, especially in work settings such as the UK's National Health Service (NHS). It is therefore important to address the particular issues and considerations that arise whilst providing EMDR supervision in groups.

Why group supervision?

The most obvious reason for proving supervision in a group setting is that of economies of both time and money. Where there exists an insufficient number of EMDR Consultants, as is currently the case in the UK, group supervision rather than individual supervision is a better use of their time. In addition, the costs are less for the organisation or for the individual, if they are funding the supervision themselves. However, there are other advantages to group supervision (Bernard & Goodyear, 2019) which I have summarised here:

- Through group supervision, each supervisee has access to a wider range of practice and will learn about the utilisation of EMDR with many more clients than their own.

DOI: 10.4324/9781003214588-10

- The group format provides a much greater variety of learning experiences, for example, reflecting on the practice of colleagues.
- Each group member will benefit from a greater diversity of perspectives on their clinical work.
- The group format enables the supervisor to obtain a more comprehensive picture of their supervisee as they observe how they interact with other members of the group.
- The supervisee will learn more about how they are seen by others, which can be valuable information when considering, in supervision, the "Fourth Eye" in the Seven-Eyed model.
- The supervisee gains the opportunity to learn supervision skills, especially relevant for supervisees who are training to become Consultants themselves.
- Supervisees' experiences are normalised, finding, for example, that other EMDR therapists have the same doubts and anxieties as their own.

However, Bernard and Goodyear do also outline some of the disadvantages of group supervision:

- Particular individuals may not get what they need from supervision and the supervisee may have particular issues that the supervisor can only manage in an individual setting.
- There may be concerns about confidentiality relating to both client information and supervisees' own issues.
- The form and structure of group supervision does not mirror the practice being supervised, namely individual one-to-one therapy which is how EMDR is usually delivered.
- Certain group phenomena, such as competitiveness and insensitivity to cultural differences, can impede learning.

On balance, however, group supervision is generally found to be as effective as individual supervision (Ögren, Boëthius, & Sundin, 2014) and the advantages tend to outweigh the limitations (Bernard & Goodyear, 2019).

Types of groups

Before setting up a supervision group, one needs to consider what type of group one will be running. This will depend on a number of factors including:

- the developmental stage of the supervisees in terms of their experience of EMDR
- the demands of the context in which the group has been set up
- the time pressures and demands of each particular group meeting

Proctor and Inskipp (2001) outlined a typology for group supervision. They describe four types of supervision groups, the first three being supervisor-led groups whilst the fourth one is described as a peer group.

- Type 1: Authoritative Group (Supervision *in* a group)
- Type 2: Participative Group (Supervision *with* the group)
- Type 3: Co-operative Group (Supervision *by* the group)
- Type 4: Peer group

Type 1: Authoritative group (Supervision in a group)

The supervisor provides supervision to each supervisee in turn whilst the other supervisees are primarily observers and learners during this process. In other words, it is, in effect, individual supervision with an audience.

Type 2: Participative group (Supervision with the group)

The supervisor still takes prime responsibility for supervising each therapist. However, the supervisor also actively directs group members to co-supervise each other and comment upon each other's presentations.

Type 3: Co-operative group (Supervision by the group)

Here it is the group itself which is providing the supervision. The supervisor's role is as a facilitator and supervision monitor. In the context of EMDR supervision, it should be noted that the supervisor must still take responsibility for ensuring that comments by members of the group are in accordance with EMDR protocols. In addition, as an evaluator in relation to accreditation, the supervisor will also be assessing the group members in terms of their understand of the protocol during this process.

Type 4: Peer group

In this type of group, no individual is taking on the responsibility of supervisor. Although one individual may act as chair or coordinator (a role which might revolve around the group) this person holds no responsibility as a supervisor. Such groups exist in some regions of the UK under the auspices of the EMDR Association UK. It should be noted that peer group supervision cannot be counted towards accreditation even if there is an EMDR Consultant present at the meeting. In order to be absolutely clear about this, a decision was made by the EMDR Association UK to describe such groups as "Peer *Support* Groups" rather than "Peer Supervision Groups."

So how do we decide which kind of group to set up? Given the factors summarised above, one must first consider the developmental stage of the therapists one is supervising. If, for example, the therapists have not yet completed their basic 7/8-day training in EMDR or have only recently completed it, an Authoritative Group might be the most effective format as trainees will still be learning basic EMDR protocols and would be floundering if they were expected to comment upon each other's cases. However, in my experience, even with such groups, an element of a Participative Group can often be valuable, and I would not preclude other members of the group from commenting when one of their colleagues is presenting a case. Generally speaking, however, one would expect that, the more experienced one's supervisees are, the more appropriate it will be to run a Participative or Co-operative Group. In particular, if the group consists mainly of Consultants or Consultants-in-training, a Co-operative Group will assist them in learning and practising the skills of supervision.

A second consideration would be the context in which the group has been set up. If, for example, the group has been commissioned and funded by an organisation that employs the supervisees, and the contract explicitly specifies the way in which supervision will be conducted, it may be necessary to stick to running an Authoritative Group.

A third consideration relates to time pressures. If, for example, the group normally works Co-operatively but, on a particular occasion, the supervisees have a greater than usual number of cases to discuss, there simply may not be sufficient time to involve the whole group in discussing each case and the group may need to resort to becoming an Authoritative one for that particular meeting.

So any one group may vary between the three first types from one meeting to the next depending on the various demands of the day. In addition, a session might start in a focused way as an Authoritative Group, looking at several specific and technical questions that supervisees have brought and then, in the half-hour broaden into a Participative or Co-operative Group for a more open discussion about a general issue brought by one of the participants.

How many in the group?

The "Goldilocks" range (not too large, not too small) for a supervision group appears to be four to six members. Boalt Boëthius and Ögren (2001) say that a group of just three individuals can become too competitive whereas a group of four can relate to each other in dyads. However, as the size increases, reticent members will fail to contribute and some members may tend to dominate.

In addition, the "Guidelines regarding frequency and quantity of EMDR supervision" of the UK's EMDR Association (EMDR Association UK,

2019) (the first version of which was drafted by me) specifies a recommended group size of no more than six.

Homogeneous versus heterogeneous

There are a number of ways in which individual members of a group may differ in terms, say, of age, gender, race, nationality, professional training, and experience. In general, a more heterogeneous group functions better (Ögren et al., 2014). However, I am concerned here in thinking about the individual's level of development as an EMDR therapist as outlined in Chapter 3 in terms of Developmental Models of supervision.

What are the pros and cons of having more heterogeneity in a supervision group in terms of the EMDR development of its members? The advantage of a homogeneous group is that everyone is working at a similar level and any teaching in relation to the EMDR protocol is likely to be relevant to all the members of the group. If it is an advanced group of trainee EMDR Consultants, the group can also address issues regarding supervision which would not be relevant to those who are not yet accredited Practitioners. I have run such homogeneous groups, one for recently trained EMDR therapists working towards Practitioner accreditation and one for those working towards Consultant accreditation and both worked well.

However, I also ran a very mixed group which included trainee Consultants and those who had not yet completed their basic EMDR training. This group also worked very well and, in fact, the Consultants-in-training were able to practise and demonstrate their group supervision skills whilst I was observing them in a form of live supervision-of-supervision (see Chapter 12) which worked well for everyone.

The group context

> I have a particular supervision group based in NHS secondary care where members are carrying a lot of risk, have significant personal stuff happening, with a high level of turnover of staff, all of which impacts in the supervision group experience. (EMDR Consultant)

Given that it is a requirement that clinicians are already trained and experienced mental health professionals before embarking on EMDR training, it will be unusual for group supervision to be part of a basic therapist training course.

The main exception to this is when group supervision takes place during the Parts 2 and 3 basic training in EMDR therapy. In this context, supervision will occur amongst a group who may have no prior contact with each other, and the life of the group may be no more than two or three sessions over the course of a two-day training. In this situation, there is little opportunity for any group cohesion to take place. The group will most likely be an "Authoritative Group" and is unlikely to move beyond a "Participative Group" at best. It should also be noted that such a group will be very homogeneous in that they are exactly at the same stage of their training. In addition, such groups will, of necessity, be much larger than the ideal size, with up to 12 individuals in each group.

Another context is what Proctor (2008) refers to as an "agency group," in other words a group which has been set up by an organisation in order to provide supervision to their own employees. There is a great variation between agencies in terms of their expectations of what will occur in supervision and the amount of feedback that they require in relation to the activities and outcomes of the supervision group. An EMDR Consultant, particularly one who is being bought in from outside the organisation, needs to familiarise themselves with agency policies and to be absolutely clear about what will be expected of them.

By contrast, a "freelance group" (Proctor, 2008) may include participants who themselves are self-employed and work independently as well as those who are employed by an organisation. The supervisor has much more control about the kind of group that they wish to run and what will be expected of the group. The supervisor will also be able to specify the degree of heterogeneity of the group.

We also need to highlight the differences between a pre-existing group and a group that is created by the supervisor. As an EMDR Consultant, I have worked with pre-existing groups who all have a close working relationship prior to meeting me. I needed to learn to understand their group climate and how they functioned as a group before I could start supervising them (Hawkins & McMahon, 2020). I may also need to learn their shared language and their "in-jokes" in order to join with the group. I am the outsider, and the group will need to decide how much to let me in. In a couple of groups that I have supervised, the manager of the group was also an EMDR therapist themselves and therefore a member of the group which, itself, brought in additional dynamics.

Contrast this with a group that I have assembled myself in which it is my role to create the climate for the group and model for its members the ways in which they might interact with each other to maximise educational possibilities. In the groups I have organised myself, I have made sure that tea or coffee and food are provided, especially during the early stages of the group. This helps to "break the ice" and helps individuals to feel nurtured by the group. At the first session, I have also asked each group member to describe a case which has actually gone well for them and for which they do not need any help, in order that they have the experience of sharing something with the group in a context where they do not need to feel too vulnerable.

Organisation and structuring of groups

For group supervision to work effectively, the set-up needs to be considerably more structured than would be necessary for individual supervision. As well as ensuring that everyone's supervision needs are met by the group, the organising and structuring of the group should ensure that supervisees feel safe enough to share their vulnerability about their struggles in working with particular clients.

Proctor (2008) describes this using a metaphor of nesting frogs. She was once given a gift of "Russian frogs" (rather than dolls) and therefore describes the following hierarchy of nesting "frogs":

- Overall contract
- Group working agreement
- Session agenda
- Minute-to-minute response management

Let us look at each of these in turn.

Overall contract

As I understand it, the contract will be the agreement that was made prior to the group even commencing. For work with an agency, this might consist of a written contract, which will specify what will be delivered and, if the supervisor is an external provider, the remuneration arrangements.

Group working agreement

This is the agreement made between the supervisor and group when it first meets. Functional arrangements will include agreements on the following:

- Time
- Place
- Time management
- Arriving and attendance
- Time allocated to each supervisee
- Reflecting on work and progress
- Note-keeping

In addition, interpersonal ground rules need to be established such as:

- Confidentiality
- Respect

The group will also need to agree on individual learning agendas for each supervisee. For EMDR therapists, examples of the issues that they may wish to focus on are:

- Developing confidence in starting the Desensitisation phase
- How to help my client find the correct NC
- When and how to deliver Interweaves

Session agenda

Proctor's third "frog" is the setting of the agenda at the start of each session. With individual supervisees we can afford to be more relaxed about this. But in group supervision it needs to be clear what the group needs to have covered before leaving time and to make sure that each individual's supervision needs have been met as far as possible. It is therefore necessary to go around the whole group to check what they wish to bring to supervision and to ascertain and clarify what the Supervision Question (SQ) is for each client to be presented. This must be done quite tightly as there can be a tendency for a supervisee to launch into providing detailed information at this stage. Supervisees will need to learn the discipline of being succinct and providing just the necessary amount of information. Here I am reminded of the letter sent by Mark Twain which started with the words: "I apologize for such a long letter – I didn't have time to write a short one."

This stage is also important in relation to the more reticent supervisees who repeatedly say, "I don't have anything to bring this week. I'll be fine just listening." It is best to make time for these people anyway, and say, "I'll give you a chance later in case anything comes up as you listen to the others." They often think of a question. In addition, the supervisor may need to start probing a little more deeply to find out why the supervisee is not bringing material to the supervision session.

In individual supervision, the management of the available time is largely the responsibility of the supervisee. They decide what they wish to bring to supervision, in what order the cases are presented and how much time they wish to spend on each case. In group supervision it is clearly the responsibility of the supervisor to be the time manager in order to ensure that the supervision needs of every member of the group have been met as far as possible.

Minute-to-minute response management

"The littlest frog – the heart of the matter: So, finally to the central management task, to which all other tasks are servant. Each individual piece of supervision (of client work or related professional issue) is what the group is about" (Proctor, 2008, p. 66).

In EMDR supervision this will start with a reiteration of the SQ which should set the scene for the presentation and the group's hopefully adaptive response to the supervisee's current dilemma.

Below I will describe a particular protocol that I have devised in order to engage the whole group in addressing the SQ.

Protocol for EMDR group supervision

As I have already mentioned several times in this book, we learn more from our mistakes than from our successes. The genesis of this protocol is a good example of this. In 2014, I attended a course on group supervision run by Robin Shohet (Shohet, 2014). It was an excellent course, and I was so enthused by Shohet's model for running a supervision group that I tried this out at a Consultants' Training run by Sandi Richman where I was teaching group supervision. Well, the group went disastrously wrong and, instead of addressing issues regarding EMDR, it quickly dissolved into examining the personal issues of members of the group including myself. I can still recall the look on Sandi's face as she became increasingly alarmed as to what was happening!

It was clear that Shohet's protocol was not going to work in the context of EMDR supervision. But, using some of the principles of his protocol, I decided to think about how I could create something more structured (as indeed the EMDR Standard Protocol is itself) whilst allowing the same kind of creative free-association process to occur as happens in EMDR therapy. I therefore came up with the following protocol in 2015 which I have since used in several EMDR Consultants' trainings and other workshops on EMDR supervision. Although it is not a protocol that I would usually use in its purest form in my everyday work, many of those who have attended my workshops have been enthused by this protocol and have told me that it helped them to really understand how one can draw in the whole group in EMDR supervision.

This protocol is appropriate for supervision groups in which supervisees are already experienced EMDR practitioners, preferably already Accredited. It should be regarded as a Co-operative Group which uses "supervision *by* the group." The fact that it has eight phases is a coincidence!

1   *Preamble* (can be reduced or omitted at subsequent meetings of the group)
    "Today we are all supervisors. In EMDR, the protocol allows processing to occur spontaneously. Similarly, this supervision protocol should allow supervision to occur spontaneously through the interactions of members of this group. As the facilitator of this group, I will only intervene if the process becomes stuck or the group needs to learn something specific about the EMDR protocol. If I do intervene, as with a cognitive interweave in EMDR, I will attempt to say the minimum necessary in order for the process of supervision to move forward."

"In a moment I will ask one of you to volunteer a Supervision Question. Before you tell us any more about your client, I will ask members of the group what they would need to know about your client in order to help you with this Supervision Question. I will then invite the supervisee to respond with more information and ask group members to respond until the supervisee feels their question has been answered. We will then discuss what we have learned and ensure that we understand the theory that underlies this learning point."

2   Ask a member of the group to provide an SQ. (If the supervisee starts to give information about the client or the statement does not actually constitute a question, continue to prompt the supervisee until they produce an actual question.) Repeat the SQ to ensure that you have understood it correctly and everyone is clear on what the question is.

3   Ask the rest of the group: "What do we need to know in order to answer this question and help [supervisee's name]?" Make sure that everyone in the group has responded.

4   Ask supervisee to respond and provide further information. (Interrupt if the information appears irrelevant to the SQ or they are providing unnecessary detail. Remind the supervisee what information the group needs in order to help them answer their question.)

5   Ask group members to comment upon the information provided. This might involve asking further questions, ideas about the formulation or possible ways forward with the therapy. If the issue is an emotional/relational one rather than a technical one, ask, "what are people feeling/noticing/experiencing right now?"

6   Repeat 3, 4, and 5 until the supervisee appears to have resolved their issue and indicates that their SQ has been answered.

7   Check with supervisee that they feel their question has been answered and they know where they are going with this particular client.

8   Summarise what has been learned. Outline the theory behind what has been learned.

As a general rule, do not comment unless:

- you are sure that no one else in the group knows the answer
- a group member's comment is off-protocol
- a group member's comment is inappropriately critical
- you are running out of time

Think of your intervention as a cognitive interweave i.e. "stay out of the way" if the process is working well and only intervene if things become stuck or go off course.

Brushing up on the protocol

As previously stated, it is often our role as EMDR supervisors to do some basic teaching about the Standard Protocol (or some other protocol) when it becomes apparent that there is a gap in the supervisee's knowledge or understanding of a particular aspect. Clearly in a group situation it will be the whole group that one will be teaching. In a heterogeneous group, it may be a good idea to ask the more experienced members of the group to explain concepts to others, which will also help the more experienced people to clarify their own understanding. As I have found from my own experience, one of the best ways of learning is by teaching (Cohen, Kulik, & Kulik, 1982).

EMDR accreditation

Obviously, the process of assessing and signing off a supervisee for accreditation purposes may not be as straightforward in a group setting as in an individual setting. Firstly, the requirement to observe the supervisee's work by video recording may need to occur outside the group if such observation will not necessarily benefit the rest of the group. In addition, there may be issues that the supervisor needs to address with a supervisee in relation to their accreditation that are not appropriate to discuss in the group setting.

I have addressed this myself in a number of ways. In one group that I supervised in an NHS service, two individuals had reached the stage of Practitioner accreditation at the same time, and I had a separate meeting with them both in order to discuss issues regarding accreditation. In a private group, set up by myself, I created a 12-month package designed to take recently trained supervisees to the stage of Practitioner accreditation. As my advertising for this group explained:

> The group will consist of 11 monthly 2-hour group sessions (leaving out August) together with an additional 4 hours of individual supervision (to be slotted in between the group sessions) in which we would focus on specific skills and areas that individuals would need to work on in order to satisfy the criteria for accreditation. So, each supervisee would have a total of 26 hours of supervision over the course of 12 months.

As far as Consultant accreditation is concerned the group setting affords some advantages. One requirement is that the supervisor has observed the trainee Consultant providing group supervision. With a couple of supervisees who have been members of a group that I have supervised, I have been able to observe their supervision of the group in-vivo as part of one of our regular group meetings.

Group dynamics

It might be argued that, in an EMDR supervision group, which is likely to be more structured than other supervision groups, issues of group dynamics are likely to be less relevant. However, what occurs between members of the group has the potential to either disrupt the functioning of the group or, conversely, increase its efficacy. Many readers will already be familiar with the best-known model of group processes described by Tuckman (Tuckman, 1965; Tuckman & Jensen, 1977) which describes five stages in the development of groups as follows:

- Forming
- Storming
- Norming
- Performing
- Adjourning

Forming (testing and dependence)

At this stage, the scene is being set for the kind of group that it will be. The supervisor will be negotiating a contract and structure for the group and will be facilitating the group in starting to become comfortable with one another.

Storming (intragroup conflict)

This is the stage at which competitiveness between group members will be at its strongest and there may be a struggle for power in the group. It has been suggested by Jacobs et al. (2015) that this stage is not always evident and may, in any event, reflect aspects of poor group leadership in setting up the group. "The effect of paying insufficient attention to the forming process can be to precipitate the group into normlessness" (Proctor, 2008, p. 96) and it is the leader's job to renegotiate how the group will function.

Norming (development and group cohesion)

In this stage, the group starts to form its own unwritten rules for how to behave in the group and a group culture is being created.

Performing (functional role-relatedness)

"When the group moves successfully into working as an engaged group, it is harvest time" (Proctor, 2008, p. 97). This is regarded as the group's most productive stage where most of the focus is on the task of supervision.

Adjourning

The group prepares to terminate, and the focus is on group members saying goodbye to one another.

As EMDR therapists we are aware that, before we can start processing a trauma, our client needs to be in a place of security and have sufficient resources in situ. Without that firm "foot in the present," they will not be ready to put their "foot in the past." Similarly with group supervision, before our supervisees will feel comfortable in sharing their vulnerabilities regarding their clinical work, they must feel safe and secure in the group and with their supervisor.

The experience of being in a supervision group and sharing our mistakes and vulnerabilities as therapists can foster a sense of shame. It is important, as a supervisor, to foster a climate in which we can be open about our vulnerabilities without feeling judged by members of the group. Whilst remaining strong and dependable as a group leader, sharing some of our own vulnerabilities and examples of when we ourselves have "messed up" as therapist should help to create the right culture in the group.

Group members need to feel a sense of security and know that they can trust other group members as well as the supervisor (Ögren, Apelman, & Klawitter, 2002). It needs to be acknowledged that some group members may re-enact previous patterns and roles from their earlier experiences in groups such as the classroom or family (Cooper & Gustafson, 1985).

Conclusion

Clinical supervision is a very complex activity, and it becomes considerably more complex in a group context. However, my own experience of doing EMDR supervision in groups is that I have found it rewarding and energising. With the right considerations and necessary structure, group supervision can become a powerful and stimulating experience for all.

Bernard, J. M., & Goodyear, R. K. (2019). *Fundamentals of clinical supervision* (6th ed.). New York, NY: Pearson.

Boalt Boëthius, S., & Ögren, M.-L. (2001). Role patterns in group supervision. *The Clinical Supervisor, 19*, 45–69.

Cohen, P. A., Kulik, J. A., & Kulik, C.-L. C. (1982). Educational outcomes of tutoring: A meta-analysis of findings. *American Educational Research Journal, 19*(2), 237–248.

Cooper, L., & Gustafson, J. P. (1985). Supervision in a group: An application of group theory. *The Clinical Supervisor, 3*(2), 7–25.

EMDR Association UK. (2019). Guidelines regarding frequency and quantity of EMDR supervision. Retrieved from website of EMDR Association UK.

Hawkins, P., & McMahon, A. (2020). *Supervision in the helping professions* (5th ed.). London: Open University Press.

Jacobs, E. E., Schimmel, C. J., Masson, R. L., & Harvill, R. L. (2015). *Group counseling: Strategies and skills.* Boston, MA: Cengage Learning.

Ögren, M.-L., Apelman, A., & Klawitter, M. (2002). The group in psychotherapy supervision. *The Clinical Supervisor, 20*(2), 147–175.

Ögren, M.-L., Boëthius, S. B., & Sundin, E. (2014). Challenges and possibilities in group supervision. In C. E. Watkins Jr & D. Milne (Eds.), *The Wiley international handbook of clinical supervision* (pp. 648–669). Chichester, UK: Wiley.

Proctor, B. (2008). *Group supervision. A guide to creative practice* (2nd ed.). London: Sage.

Proctor, B., & Inskipp, F. (2001). Group supervision. In J. Scaife (Ed.), *Supervision in the mental health professions. A practioner's guide* (pp. 99–121). London: Brunner-Routledge.

Shohet, R. (2014). *Group supervision course, CSTD,* London.

Tuckman, B. W. (1965). Developmental sequence in small groups. *Psychological Bulletin, 63*(6), 384.

Tuckman, B. W., & Jensen, M. A. C. (1977). Stages of small-group development revisited. *Group & Organization Studies, 2*(4), 419–427.

Chapter 10

The mechanics of supervision

- Online supervision
- Media for observing EMDR therapy
- Recording therapy sessions

Online supervision

I am old enough to recall a time when the only way of doing supervision was for two individuals to sit in a room together. The whole supervisory process would take place only in this context, from the initial meeting and contracting to the sessions themselves.

Even before the Covid-19 pandemic, online supervision was becoming widespread. Well before the pandemic, a chapter by Rousmaniere (2014) described the extensive use of technologies to deliver supervision in many therapeutic modalities, including EMDR, in what he described as "technology-assisted supervision and training" (TAST). Other terms that have been used are "cybersupervision," "web-based training," "telemedicine," "telehealth," "computer-based learning," "computer-assisted learning," "technology-assisted distance supervision and consultation," "e-learning," and "computer-mediated training" (Rousmaniere, 2014).

Five years later, a review of the literature by Inman et al. (2019) concluded that in-person supervision and live teleconferencing supervision (i.e. face-to-face over the Internet) were equally effective. Supervisees reported that technology, specifically e-mail technology, allowed for more ongoing access to their supervisors and the use of e-mail allowed them to clarify their thoughts before responding to supervisors, which would not be possible with in-person supervision. Other reported advantages were greater convenience and flexibility in scheduling meetings, an increased sense of connectedness, and reduced feelings of isolation. Telesupervision appeared to allow supervisees to stay on task, and to access and express emotions clearly and readily. In addition, it also allowed supervisees and supervisors from different countries to gain varying cultural perspectives.

However, on the downside, Inman et al concluded that telesupervision impeded supervisees' involvement with supervision. Initially, due to

DOI: 10.4324/9781003214588-11

security concerns, some supervisees reported that they were less present and less open in supervision. Specifically, they indicated that they were concerned that the content of supervision sessions might not be as confidential. However, after gaining more confidence and comfort with the technology, students' fear diminished, and their attitudes toward distance supervision also seemed to improve. The most common supervisee complaints were delays in responses due to technology glitches although one study revealed that, despite technical issues, the problems did not negatively impact the overall supervision experience for supervisees (Inman, Soheilian, & Luu, 2019).

Belšak and Simonič (2018) raised additional concerns, stating that, following professional associations' codes of ethics and legal regulations, the supervisor and supervisee should first consider how to protect the confidentiality of clients when processing, transmitting, storing, and archiving their personal data. They pointed out that the supervision informed-consent process should also include information on all technology used, including steps taken to protect the client.

A more recent article by Phillips et al. (2021) looks at the impact of the Covid-19 pandemic on the use of telesupervision and the understandable increase in its use since 2020. They speculate that telesupervision practice would certainly continue beyond the pandemic. They point out that there is some evidence that prior in-person experience with a supervisor is beneficial for telesupervision (Martin, Lizarondo, & Kumar, 2018) but also some evidence that this might not be necessary (Jordan & Shearer, 2019; Tarlow et al., 2020). They also wonder whether prior in-person contact is more important for early practicum trainees (with relatively limited clinical skills and confidence), as compared to postdoctoral residents (with more advanced competence and associated confidence).

Inman et al. (2019) provided a case study on cross-cultural telesupervision. They noted that technology can lead to challenges but also increased availability of cross-cultural experiences. They recommend that in telesupervision experiences, supervisors engage in "multicultural discussions" (p. 404) and should remain mindful of context, both supervisor and trainee identities, power differentials, and working alliance.

In conclusion then, it appears that online supervision or telesupervision is here to stay and that, generally speaking, it is at least as effective as in-person supervision.

Media for observing EMDR therapy

The EMDR Europe criteria for accreditation as an EMDR Practitioner states that "the EMDR Clinical Supervisor supervising your application has directly witnessed your EMDR work either on video or In Vivo." For Consultant accreditation, it states that the supervisor has "witnessed a minimum of three videos, or in-vivo sessions meeting the required standard, of the applicant's professional practice of which one must be clinical, the second of them providing individual EMDR clinical supervision and the third of them providing Group EMDR clinical supervision" (EMDR Association UK, 2022).

This need for our therapy and supervision to be observed is a requirement for accreditation in Europe (although not in North America) and such observation is often prompted by such a need. However, it is important to acknowledge that having one's work observed is as much a part of the Educating function of supervision as it is an aspect of the Evaluating function.

In a section entitled, "Evidence to determine competency in EMDR therapy," Farrell (2020) describes five different media for observing EMDR therapy as follows:

- Verbal reports
- Verbatim reports
- Written/Clinical documentation review
- Video recordings
- Simulation

Derek Farrell helpfully describes each of these and the advantages and disadvantages of each in a table of which I have created a modified version (Table 10.1). To Farrell's original five categories, I have added a sixth category of "In-vivo Supervision" during which the supervisor is physically present in the room, behind a one-way mirror or observing online as the therapy takes place. This is, in fact, one of the forms of observation specified in the EMDR Europe accreditation criteria as outlined above.

A similar list of pros and cons was presented by Andrew Leeds (Leeds, 2009).

Recording therapy sessions

As long ago as 1983, in his seminal paper, Bordin (1983) said "the greatest professional growth is likely to occur around review of sound or video-taped recordings of one's interviews" (p. 39). The following quote from 1997 is also relevant here:

> The word supervision is derived from the Latin *super*, meaning "over", and *videre*, "to see". In a literal sense, audio- and video-recordings provide a direct, factually correct vision of what transpired in the therapy session. It is this direct access, unfiltered through the therapist's recollections, that is the prime advantage of the recording. The patient and therapist can be heard in action, and seen if videoed, which is a very different matter from those events being reported. The simple exercise of comparing one's notes on a session with a tape-recording dramatically highlights the deficiencies of memory,

Table 10.1 A comparison of different media used for EMDR supervision

Medium	Description	Advantages	Disadvantages
Verbal reporting	• Supervisee provides verbal reports of the EMDR session • Group discussion about clinical situation	• Informal • Efficient use of time • Greater spontaneity • Supervisee controls the narrative	• The EMDR Session is seen only through the "eyes" of the supervisee • Absence of non-verbal components
Verbatim report/ Transcripts	• Written transcript of clinical sessions including both therapist and client	• See the flow and structure of the EMDR clinical session • Helps track process and orientation to the EMDR protocol • Enhances AIP case conceptualisation • Enhances recall to provide greater context • Enhances reflection • Provides accurate documentation of the EMDR session(s)	• Vital context may be missed • Can be very time-consuming • Often context maybe compromised
Written/case file documentation review	• Review of ALL the clinical documentation relating to the client, including psychometrics, other professional inputs, etc.	• Provides a more comprehensive and broader reach in understanding the client • Useful in determining compliance, safe and effective practice • Effective quality control • Ensures consistency in clinical documentation	• May not be feasible • Documentation often misses vital context • Documentation may be "sanitised" and potentially differ from what "actually" may have occurred • Essence of clinical supervision may get lost • Can very easily become case management rather than competency development

(Continued)

Table 10.1 (Continued)

Medium	Description	Advantages	Disadvantages
Video recording	• Providing a digital recording of the EMDR clinical session	• Clearly see both verbal and non-verbal exchanges between the EMDR therapist and the client • Can focus on specific EMDR skills and practice • Provides a richer context of what occurred "real time" • Potentially highlights difference between what is "declared" and what is "evidenced"	• Can be time-consuming • Need for equipment and resources • Not possible to record various client groups • Organisations/institutions may not grant permission for video recording • Requires client permission • Clarification of "ownership" of the video • Anxiety provoking and performance anxiety
Simulation	• Role play re-enactment	• Focus of the role play can be easily determined • Ability to highlight essential EMDR skills and professional development • Can be "stopped" in real-time to emphasise a specific teaching and learning point • Removes the organisational and technical dilemmas	• Potentially too reductionist • Absence of a "real life" or client context • Performance anxiety
In-vivo supervision	• Live supervision by the supervisor as the therapy session takes place (supervisor in the room, behind a screen or live online)	• Clearly see both verbal and non-verbal exchanges between the EMDR therapist and the client • Supervisor can intervene in real-time if the supervisee gets stuck or asks for assistance	• Can be time-consuming • Presence of the supervisor may affect client/therapist relationship • Requires client permission • Anxiety provoking and performance anxiety

Source: Based upon a table in an online presentation by Derek Farrell on Advanced clinical supervision and consultation skills in enhancing competency in EMDR therapy in 2020.

especially when emotionally-charged and complex issues are emerging and being explored. In recollection, whole segments of interaction are not recorded in memory, the sequence of interactions become reordered, key statements by the patient are either misheard or not heard, elements are magnified or diminished, and interpretations take on a wishful perfection.

(Aveline, 1997, p. 82)

What are the advantages of recording our therapy sessions for the purpose of supervision? The main reason for doing so relates to the inadequacy of alternatives. Most supervision is based on verbal reporting. "Many supervisors who rely on self-report have fallen into stagnation ... at its worst, self-report is a method whereby supervisees *distort* (rather than *report*) their work, even if they are not consciously doing so" (Bernard & Goodyear, 2019, p. 164). Muslin et al. (1981) found that 54% of the themes of video-taped interviews were not reported in supervision and some degree of distortion was present in 54% of the interviews. Ladany et al. (1996) reported that 97% of supervisees were conscious of keeping relevant material out of their supervision.

For a therapy such as EMDR which has a clear, structured procedure, it is particularly important that the supervisor has an opportunity to observe their supervisee's work in order to be sure that they are adhering to the EMDR protocol. In my own experience, many surprises have occurred when I have viewed my supervisee's videos. One of my supervisees had always impressed me with his competence and grasp of the EMDR protocol and I assumed that viewing one of his videos would just be a formality. Indeed, when I observed the video, his cognitive interweaves were most creative and innovative. Unfortunately, however, he did not need to use them at all because the client was processing quite spontaneously. Another supervisee always seemed confused and muddled during supervision so I was rather dreading what her video recording would look like. To my surprise, I observed a competent and apparently confident therapist using the protocol very effectively. I realised that her persona in supervision was, perhaps, a response to the power relationship that existed in that setting and it bore little relationship to how she presented as a therapist.

Once our supervisee has produced a video, what is the best way of viewing it? In order to make a decision about this, we need to bear in mind the dual roles of the Educating and Evaluating functions of supervision. In terms of the Educating function, it might be best to ask the supervisee to choose which sections of the video they wish to present at the points where they were struggling or uncertain as to how to proceed. In terms of the Evaluating function which we require for accreditation, it might be better for the supervisor to watch a whole therapy session at some other time and subsequently provide feedback to the supervisee at the next supervision session. Whilst this affords less opportunity for discussion, instant feedback and learning, it is more economical of time.

As well as those described in the relevant box above, Scaife (2019) points out a number of disadvantages of recording therapy sessions. Firstly, the recording of the session may affect the degree of empathy between the client and therapist. She says that "the presence of a third ear or eye can be perceived as inhibiting, leading to an awkwardness and reticence on the part of either or both parties" (p. 218). To counter this from my own experience, I would agree with Urdang (1999) that the active involvement of the client in deciding whether to record will offset the potential intrusion into the therapeutic relationship.

A second potential disadvantage outlined by Scaife is one of self-consciousness. People are generally critical of how they look or sound on seeing themselves on video. She suggests that practitioner experiment by recording themselves in a non-clinical setting until they become accustomed to this experience.

Thirdly, Scaife warns against the therapist becoming anxious or defensive whilst being recorded. Topor et al. (2017) outline ways in which such performance anxiety can be reduced:

- Build a positive, collaborative, trusting learner-supervisor relationship.
- Establish a learning contract for supervision.
- Expose learners to the video recording equipment and process early in training.
- Discuss strategies to introduce video recording to patients.
- Use learning theory and a developmentally appropriate supervisory framework.
- Directly address anxiety related to using video recording with the learner.
- Identify cognitive and behavioural strategies for learners to manage their anxiety (being careful not to engage in psychotherapy with the learner).
- Show supervisors' own video recordings conducting psychotherapy.
- Explore the possibility of small group supervision.

Scaife's fourth concern relates to confidentiality, consent and security. She points out the importance of the client being able to provide properly informed consent and that security of the records is extremely important to ensure. Aveline (1997) stated that being recorded may be experienced as abusive by some clients who, in certain cases may feel unable to refuse consent to being recorded as a result of abuse and coercion earlier in their life. It would certainly be important to be aware of such issues when deciding whether to request consent to recording with particular clients.

Scaife's fifth and last concern is in relation to technical skills and, in particular, getting a recording that is audible. However, with advancing technology and the fact that most therapists will carry a video recording device with them in the form of a smartphone, such issues are likely to become less pressing.

I have to admit that, for me, perhaps, having my work observed feels like second nature. I come from a family of classical musicians and have always known that, to learn a musical instrument, you have to play in front of your teacher. For many others, however, the experience of having your work observed will be much harder and there is often the fear of shame attached to showing oneself at work. This may be an issue in itself that needs to be addressed in supervision. Neufeldt et al. (1996) found that a willingness to experience vulnerability was a necessary quality in relation to agreeing to use recordings of therapy sessions. Scaife (2019) suggests that the supervisor should share their own willingness to show their vulnerability by letting clients see recordings of their own work. Tony Rousmaniere, one of the big names in clinical supervision research, "starts each training year by showing his trainees a clip of a video in which he forgets the client's name" (Bernard & Goodyear, 2019, p. 167). Some of the videos of my own work which I present in trainings have several protocol mistakes and I use this as a teaching exercise during the training to "spot Robin's mistakes."

Scaife also suggests that we should discuss with reluctant supervisees "when, rather than if, they wish to experience recorded or live supervision of their work" (Scaife, 2019, p. 209). One excuse offered by supervisees relates to consent and their assertion that their clients would be uncomfortable about the recording of sessions. Perhaps we should tell them about the study by Briggie et al. (2016) who found that 52% of clients expressed no or slight concerns and 71% were willing to consider audio or video recording. It has certainly been my own experience and that of my supervisees that, once you pluck up the courage to ask your clients about recording sessions, most clients will be in agreement. I would share with my supervisees that it can be scary to ask and that I have found this to be scary myself. But once you get into the habit of asking, you will be surprised by the positive response.

Conclusion

The medium by which EMDR supervision is provided is crucial in terms of all three functions of supervision. Of particular importance is having one's work observed, either through a video recording or in vivo. Supervisees will learn much more about their own practice and how it can be enhanced if their supervisor can observe them at work. They will feel supported and enabled, and most importantly of all, the supervisor will be able to accurately evaluate their supervisee's adherence to the EMDR protocol for the purposes of accreditation.

Aveline, M. (1997). The use of audiotapes in supervision of psychotherapy. In G. Shipton (Ed.), *Supervision of psychotherapy and counseling: Making a place to think* (pp. 80–92). Buckingham, UK: Open University Press.

Belšak, K., & Simonič, A. (2018). Ethical issues in the use of technology in clinical supervision. *Psihoterapija, 32*(2), 233–246.

Bernard, J. M., & Goodyear, R. K. (2019). *Fundamentals of clinical supervision* (6th ed.). New York, NY: Pearson.

Bordin, E. S. (1983). A working alliance based model of supervision. *The Counseling Psychologist, 11*(1), 35–42.

Briggie, A. M., Hilsenroth, M. J., Conway, F., Muran, J. C., & Jackson, J. M. (2016). Patient comfort with audio or video recording of their psychotherapy sessions: Relation to symptomatology, treatment refusal, duration, and outcome. *Professional Psychology: Research and Practice, 47*(1), 66.

EMDR Association UK. (2022). EMDR Europe Consultant Competency Based Framework.

Farrell, D. (2020). *Advanced clinical supervision and consultation skills in enhancing competency in EMDR therapy.* EMDR Lebanon Association.

Inman, A. G., Bashian, H., Pendse, A. C., & Luu, L. P. (2019). Publication trends in telesupervision: A content analysis study. *The Clinical Supervisor, 38*(1), 97–115.

Inman, A. G., Soheilian, S. S., & Luu, L. P. (2019). Telesupervision: Building bridges in a digital era. *Journal of Clinical Psychology, 75*(2), 292–301.

Jordan, S. E., & Shearer, E. M. (2019). An exploration of supervision delivered via clinical video telehealth (CVT). *Training and Education in Professional Psychology, 13*(4), 323.

Ladany, N., Hill, C. E., Corbett, M. M., & Nutt, E. A. (1996). Nature, extent, and importance of what psychotherapy trainees do not disclose to their supervisors. *Journal of Counseling Psychology, 43*(1), 10.

Leeds, A. (2009). *How to use work samples and case documentation in remote EMDR Consultation.* Paper presented at the 20th EMDRIA Conference, Atlanta.

Martin, P., Lizarondo, L., & Kumar, S. (2018). A systematic review of the factors that influence the quality and effectiveness of telesupervision for health professionals. *Journal of Telemedicine and Telecare, 24*(4), 271–281.

Muslin, H. L., Thurnblad, R. J., & Meschel, G. (1981). The fate of the clinical interview: An observational study. *The American Journal of Psychiatry, 138*, 822–825.

Neufeldt, S. A., Karno, M. P., & Nelson, M. L. (1996). A qualitative study of experts' conceptualizations of supervisee reflectivity. *Journal of Counseling Psychology, 43*(1), 3.

Phillips, L. A., Logan, J. N., & Mather, D. B. (2021). COVID-19 and beyond: Telesupervision training within the supervision competency. *Training and Education in Professional Psychology, 15*(4), 284–289.

Rousmaniere, T. (2014). Using technology to enhance clinical supervision and training. In C. Watkins, & D. Milne (Eds.), *The Wiley international handbook of clinical supervision* (pp. 204–237). Chichester, UK: Wiley.

Scaife, J. (2019). *Supervision in clinical practice: a practitioner's guide* (3rd ed.). Milton Park, Abingdon, Oxon: Routledge.

Tarlow, K. R., McCord, C. E., Nelon, J. L., & Bernhard, P. A. (2020). Comparing in-person supervision and telesupervision: A multiple baseline single-case study. *Journal of Psychotherapy Integration, 30*(2), 383.

Topor, D. R., AhnAllen, C. G., Mulligan, E. A., & Dickey, C. C. (2017). Using video recordings of psychotherapy sessions in supervision: Strategies to reduce learner anxiety. *Academic Psychiatry, 41*(1), 40–43.

Urdang, E. (1999). The video lab: Mirroring reflections of self and the other. *The Clinical Supervisor, 18*(2), 143–164.

Chapter 11

Facilitation at EMDR trainings

- Learning a new model
- Live supervision and the "reflecting team"
- Deliberate practice
- Guidelines for facilitators

For many readers of this book, this chapter may not be relevant. However, the role of the Facilitator on EMDR basic trainings is, of itself, a particular kind of supervision. Therefore, in my view, this deserves a separate chapter of its own.

There are two main ways in which facilitating differs from regular EMDR supervision as follows:

- Trainees are at the very beginning of utilising and experiencing EMDR. Both the "therapist" and the "client" are learning about EMDR simultaneously during the course of the EMDR practice at an EMDR training.
- The supervision is "live," in that it occurs whilst the therapy is actually taking place, rather than after the event.

Learning a new model

The AIP model can be useful in conceptualising what is happening when therapists start training in EMDR. Some trainees may already be very experienced in a particular therapeutic model and struggle to assimilate what they are learning about EMDR with what they already know and understand. Others may have some unprocessed issues relating to earlier experiences with learning a new skill. Often, this all comes to a head when they start to do their own EMDR practice during an EMDR training. Think about the AIP model as you read this extract from an oft-quoted paper by Jack Mezirow:

To facilitate transformative learning, educators must help learners become aware and critical of their own and others' assumptions. Learners need practice in recognizing frames of reference and using their imaginations to

DOI: 10.4324/9781003214588-12

redefine problems from a different perspective. Finally, learners need to be assisted to participate effectively in discourse. Discourse is necessary to validate what and how one understands, or to arrive at a best judgment regarding a belief. In this sense, learning is a social process, and discourse becomes central to making meaning. Effective discourse depends on how well the educator can create a situation in which those participating have full information; are free from coercion; have equal opportunity to assume the various roles of discourse (to advance beliefs, challenge, defend, explain, assess evidence, and judge arguments); become critically reflective of assumptions; are empathic and open to other perspectives; are willing to listen and to search for common ground or a synthesis of different points of view; and can make a tentative best judgment to guide action. These ideal conditions of discourse are also ideal conditions of adult learning and of education.

Transformative learning requires a form of education very different from that commonly associated with children. New information is only a resource in the adult learning process. To become meaningful, learning requires that new information be incorporated by the learner into an already well-developed symbolic frame of reference, an active process involving thought, feelings, and disposition. The learner may also have to be helped to transform his or her frame of reference to fully understand the experience.

(Mezirow, 1997, p. 10)

It often happens during the actual practice of EMDR in an EMDR training that the trainee, whether in the role of therapist or client, first really "gets" what EMDR is about and fully understands what a powerful therapy it can be. This is in itself a transformative experience and, as a facilitator, it is our job to, well, "facilitate" this!

However, it can also be during the EMDR practice on a training where the trainee gets stuck in their learning process. One form of "stuckness" is where, as the client, the trainee cannot think of a minor traumatic event to work on, or they do not feel there is any personal event that they are prepared to bring to the training. In my experience, if they feel unable to work on their own stuff, regardless of the reason, they will also have great difficulty in subsequently using EMDR therapy as a therapist. Such trainees will often complete the training but then never use EMDR in their practice and will retreat back to a therapy, such as CBT, which feels safer for them.

Another form of stuckness becomes apparent when the trainee assumes the role of the therapist. On several occasions I have seen what I would describe as the "rabbit in the headlights" phenomenon where the trainee appears to be paralysed and requires a great deal of prompting, for example, to get through the Assessment Phase. This will often be because they are being impacted by a previous unprocessed memory regarding a learning situation. For such trainees, it may be necessary for them to do some work on this (possibly using EMDR) in order to remove their blocking beliefs in relation to learning a new skill.

Live supervision and the "reflecting team"

In EMDR, we use the term "in-vivo supervision" to describe the supervisor observing the supervisee as they provide therapy in real-time. "Live supervision" is a type of in-vivo supervision where the supervisor is not just observing but may also be providing supervision as the therapy proceeds.

> Live supervision is a term describing the process by which someone guides the therapist while he works. The person supervising watches the session, usually behind a one-way mirror, and intrudes upon it to guide the therapist's behavior at the moment the action is happening.
>
> (Montalvo, 1973, p. 343)

Readers with a background in family therapy will be aware of the concept and practice of live supervision and the powerful impact that it can have on the therapeutic process (Maaß et al., 2022).

Although regular EMDR supervision can sometimes be "live," this is rare. When facilitating an EMDR training, however, the supervision will inevitably be live and there are particular considerations that we need to take regarding this.

Although not the purpose of supervising in this way, it is inevitable that the client will be affected by the live supervision that the trainee therapist is receiving from the facilitator. As this is occurring in a training situation, the facilitator needs to be aware that both the trainee and the client will be learning from the facilitator's interventions. This way of working has many similarities to the process of using a "reflecting team" in which the conversation that occurs between the therapist and supervisor in the presence of the client can, of itself, constitute a powerful therapeutic intervention (Andersen, 1987).

Deliberate practice

Whilst this issue is relevant to EMDR supervision in general, it is particularly pertinent to facilitation at EMDR trainings and for this reason, I am discussing it in this chapter.

There is a popular notion that, if you have practised a skill for long enough, you can become a master of that skill. Best known is the "10,000-hour rule" that suggests that after 10,000 hours of practice in any skill one can become an expert in it (Ericsson & Charness, 1994; Gladwell, 2008).

However, subsequent researchers have pointed out that this is an over-simplification. In fact, instead of improving with experience, the effectiveness of the average practitioner plateaus early on and slowly deteriorates (Miller & Hubble, 2011).

Ericsson et al. (1993) introduced the term "deliberate practice" (DP) which was elaborated upon by Miller et al. (2017). The key attribute of DP is to "seek out challenges that go beyond their current level of reliable achievement – ideally in a safe and optimal learning context that allows immediate feedback and gradual refinement by repetition" (Ericsson, 2009, p. 425). According to Miller et al. (2017), the deliberate practice framework contains four key elements:

1 A focused and systematic effort to improve performance pursued over an extended period
2 Involvement of and guidance from a coach/teacher/mentor
3 Immediate, ongoing feedback
4 Successive refinement and repetition via solo practice outside of performance

In my own trainings, I introduce the EMDR practice by reminding trainees that they will learn most from their mistakes and tell them that making mistakes is alright. Perhaps I should quote from Miller et al. (2017) as follows:

> Top-performing stand-up comedians provide an excellent example of this "error-centric" approach (Coyle, 2009). Average comedians focus on telling jokes. In contrast, headliners are not invested in any particular gag or routine. Their purpose is to entertain. To that end, they watch, observe, and listen to the audience, using audience reactions to rework, change, and nuance their material until it elicits what they are there to evoke, laughter.
>
> (Miller et al., 2017, p. 27)

What I am taking from this in relation to facilitation on an EMDR training is the evidence that the process of learning a new therapeutic skill whilst receiving live supervision is a very powerful and effective means to developing therapy skills.

Guidelines for facilitators

As an EMDR trainer, I have developed a set of practical guidelines which has evolved over time with feedback from many of my facilitators. My initial draft of these guidelines were assisted by reference to two documents (EMDR Institute, 2002; Wesson & Van Diest, n.d.).

Before the whole training starts

- Make sure you know where the toilets are – someone is bound to ask you!
- Find out how the heating and ventilation works so that you can adjust it during the training if necessary.
- Find out who needs to be contacted for technical help if this arises during the training.
- Sit in a place where you can be seen and heard in case the trainer wishes to include you when answering a question from a trainee.
- Be available to sort out manuals, badges, etc., and check in trainees as they arrive in order that the trainer can concentrate on setting up AV.

During the training

- Be aware of how trainees are. You may notice something that the trainer has not observed, for example, trainees are looking too hot or cold, are irritated by some disturbance, having difficulty hearing or are even bored! If so, alert the trainer at an appropriate time.
- Make yourself available to answer questions during the breaks.
- Offer to get the trainer a drink if they appear to be busy during a break. If you need to take a break yourself, do this during the teaching session when you are not necessarily required.
- If someone leaves the room and it appears possible that they may have been triggered by something happening in the main session, go and check in with them to find out what is going on and then encourage them to come back in.

Before the EMDR practice session starts

- Make sure that you have a list of names from the trainer of who will be in your group.
- Check with the trainer whether there are any trainees that need to be kept in different groups, for example, because one is the boss of another. Decide on the group sizes. They could be in groups of three (client, therapist and observer) but if the numbers are not divisible by three, it will be necessary to have one or two groups of two. Groups of two may be preferable to maximise the opportunity for everyone to have experienced both the role of therapist and client, but if the group is an odd number at least one group of three may be necessary.
- Checking the room: In good time before the session starts, make sure that you know the location of the room that you will be using and that it has the correct number of chairs, is at the right temperature, is sufficiently ventilated, etc. Find out how the heating can be changed if necessary.
- Obtain a supply of practice worksheets from the trainer.
- Get a supply of tissues!

At the start of the EMDR therapy first practice session

- If it is a large training where it has not been possible for everyone to introduce themselves, the facilitator can ask for introductions amongst their smaller group of 12 on the first occasion that they are together. This is also an opportunity to see if the trainees have any concerns about the practice which they were reluctant to ask about in the large group.
- Make it clear that you will be available for any small group to call you over if they are stuck or have a question. Also tell them that, in any event, you will be circulating around the groups and listening in on the session as it progresses.
- Tell them that, once the therapy has commenced, you will speak only to the therapist and not to the client or observer. This is in order that the therapeutic relationship is maintained and any intervention from the facilitator interrupts the flow of therapy as little as possible. Explain that when the group debriefs at the end, the client and observer will have a chance to speak with you directly.
- Make it clear that they are bound to make mistakes and that they are here to learn rather than try and execute a perfect therapy session. The more mistakes they make the more they will learn.

Arranging the groups in the room(s)

- Make the most of the available space so that each group is as much out of earshot from other groups as possible.
- Arrange the chairs so that the client is facing the wall and has no one in their direct line of sight. As well as ensuring that the client is not distracted, this means that the therapist will be facing into the room and it will be easier for the facilitator to communicate with them, even if they are across the room. Also, ensure that the observer is not in the client's field of vision.
- The client should not have their training manual or worksheets on their lap, nor a pen as they will be tempted to be therapist as well as client.
- Sometimes the client really struggles with the distraction of other groups being in the room. One solution is to put their fingers in their ears during processing.
- If necessary, it should be made clear to the observer that they are there to *observe*, not look around the room or check their phone!

Checking the assessment phase

- At the Part 1 training, ask trainees to call you over to check the Assessment Phase before commencing the Desensitisation Phase. Speak to the therapist and ask them to take you through the answers to each of the questions in the Assessment Phase. Give appropriate feedback if anything needs to be changed, for example, the NC is not correct.

- Make sure that the target memory is appropriate for a training session with a SUD of 6 or less.
- Before starting the Desensitisation Phase, make sure that they have tested out the preferred form of BLS, speed of eye movements, distance etc.
- Make sure that trainees are using the Assessment worksheet and using the specified wording on this sheet. Also, make sure that they have the Desensitisation worksheet in front of them and that they work from this instead of just "winging it!"

Intervening whilst a therapy session is progressing

- There are two situations in which it is appropriate to intervene during a session:

  - Invited: When you are invited to do so by the therapist because they have got stuck and have a dilemma as to how to proceed.
  - Uninvited: When you can see that things are going wrong and will become worse without your intervention. Obviously, this will be intrusive, and you first need to carefully assess whether they need an immediate intervention or whether your feedback can wait until the end of the session. Also, you need to decide on the timing of your intrusion. Usually, this would be at the end of a set, but you may decide to wait for a set or two in order to find a more opportune moment to intervene.

- In either situation, rather like a cognitive interweave, aim for minimal intervention. You can explain things in more detail at the end of the session which is the time when it might be appropriate to explain the theory behind what you briefly said during the session.
- Common interventions:

  - When processing stops because something new comes up: Encourage the therapist to "keep going and see what happens next" or prompt them with the words "just notice" and a brief wave of your arm.
  - During an abreaction, whisper words of encouragement to the therapist. This will also help the client to feel supported.
  - Tell them when they are doing well!

- In certain situations, with a therapist who is having great difficulty following the protocol, it may be necessary to initially supervise them very closely step by step. Try to keep out of the client's line of vision whilst doing so.
- As you will have explained before the session has started, speak only to the therapist and not to the client or observer. Try to position yourself as close to the therapist's ear as possible. The client and observer will hear what you are saying but you are making it clear that it is the therapist that you need to communicate with. If the client or observer speak to you or try to

engage you in conversion, explain to them that, at this moment, it will be more helpful to speak only to the therapist and you do not mean to be rude by not engaging with them.

Feedback and discussion at the end of a therapy session

If possible, make the time to speak with each group at the end of the therapy session. Make sure you have received feedback from both the therapist and client regarding their experience and that the observer has also been invited to share their observations. Answer any questions that may arise from the session. Explain any theory that may be relevant to any issues that have arisen. As much as possible, relate your feedback to what the trainer has been teaching.

"Shooshing"

Sometimes, when a group has finished their therapy session and the other groups are still continuing, the group that has finished will become louder and there may, quite understandably, be laughter, as the group debriefs and unwinds. The facilitator should be aware of this and, if necessary, ask the group to speak more softly to avoid disturbing other groups. Also, make sure there is no unnecessary roaming in and out of the room that may disturb other groups. If it is near the end of the session, you might suggest that they move outside the room.

Managing the time

- Make sure you know what time the session is due to end. Individual therapy sessions need to end in good time before the end, so you may need to prompt a group to wrap it up as an incomplete session.
- In groups of 3, make sure that the "observer" becomes the "client" or "therapist" in the next round and does not avoid doing each of the roles.
- After one hour, change over to the next couple so that one "client" does not hog the whole 2-hour practicum session.

Reporting back to the trainer

Give the trainer some general feedback about how the session went when you next have the opportunity. If you have any specific concerns about any of the trainees, mention this to the trainer.

Facilitating online

- Make sure that you visit each breakout room regularly.
- When you visit a breakout room, first ensure that your microphone and

video are both switched off in order to reduce the intrusiveness. Be aware that some trainees have described seeing a still picture of the facilitator as "spooky" so you may need to temporarily delete your photo from your Zoom account.

- Keep feedback to the trainer separate from the main Zoom call in case your comments are overheard by trainees.
- Be aware of the "chat" facility and that it may be possible to answer some questions through the chat facility.

Conclusion

In my experience, facilitating at an EMDR training can be one of the most powerful and rewarding forms of supervision as we witness our trainees discovering the "magic" of EMDR therapy for the first time. Be aware that, because the supervision is "live," whatever you say will impact on both therapist and client and that each may contextualise what you have said in a different way. Also be aware that, for some trainees, practicing a new model live, in the presence of a facilitator, can be quite triggering and overwhelming and they may need a considerable amount of support with this process.

Andersen, T. (1987). The reflecting team: Dialogue and meta-dialogue in clinical work. *Family Process*, 26(4), 415–428.

Coyle, D. (2009). *The talent code: Unlocking the secret of skill in maths, art, music, sport, and just about everything else*. London: Random House.

EMDR Institute. (2002). *Facilitator guidelines, policies and training handbook*. Watsonville, CA: EMDR Institute.

Ericsson, K. A. (2009). *Development of professional expertise: Toward measurement of expert performance and design of optimal learning environments*. Cambridge, UK: Cambridge University Press.

Ericsson, K. A., & Charness, N. (1994). Expert performance: Its structure and acquisition. *American Psychologist*, 49(8), 725.

Ericsson, K. A., Krampe, R. T., & Tesch-Römer, C. (1993). The role of deliberate practice in the acquisition of expert performance. *Psychological Review*, 100(3), 363.

Gladwell, M. (2008). *Outliers: The story of success*. New York, NY: Little, Brown.

Maaß, U., Kühne, F., Poltz, N., Lorenz, A., Ay-Bryson, D. S., & Weck, F. (2022). Live supervision in psychotherapy training—A systematic review. *Training and Education in Professional Psychology*, 16(2), 130.

Mezirow, J. (1997). Transformative learning: Theory to practice. *New Directions for Adult and Continuing Education*, 74, 5–12.

Miller, S. D., & Hubble, M. (2011). The road to mastery. *Psychotherapy Networker*, 35, 22–31.

Miller, S. D., Hubble, M., & Chow, D. (2017). Professional development: From oxymoron to reality. In T. Rousmaniere, R. Goodyear, S. Miller, & B. Wampold (Eds.), *The cycle of excellence: Using deliberate practice to improve supervision and training* (pp. 23–47). Chichester, UK: Wiley.

Montalvo, B. (1973). Aspects of live supervision. *Family Process, 12*(4), 343–359.

Wesson, M., & Van Diest, C. (n.d.). *Role of the EMDR facilitator. EMDR accredited training*. Chester, UK: EMDR Academy.

Chapter 12

Training EMDR supervisors

- Consultants training
- Supervision of supervision – "metasupervision"
- Accreditation as an EMDR Consultant

As a small child, I recall my mother telling me about a local teacher training college. I reacted with surprise and amusement that even teachers needed their *own* teachers to teach *them* how to be teachers! A young part of me is still chuckling about this as I start writing this chapter.

Stoltenberg and McNeill (2011) have adapted their Developmental model (see Chapter 3) to describe the development of the supervisor. Some of their descriptions do not fit with my own experience and understanding of supervisor development but the following aspects are, I think, relevant and useful in relation to the development of an EMDR Consultant:

- Level 1 supervisors are focused on doing the "right" thing, tending to apply a mechanistic approach to supervision and may take a strong "expert" role with their supervisees. I recall one of my EMDR Consultants in training telling me that they were trying to "be like Robin" as a supervisor. Whilst I felt flattered by this, I had to point out that they needed to develop their own style of supervision and that this would come with time. Level 1 trainee supervisors also tend to be uncomfortable and anxious about providing feedback to their supervisees.
- Level 2 supervisors are starting to realise the complexity of the supervision process. According to Stoltenberg and McNeill (2011), these trainee supervisors are best matched with a Level 1 supervisee, who is at the start of their training.
- Level 3 supervisors are more autonomous. They are as aware of their supervisees as they are of themselves and are comfortable in giving constructive critical feedback to their supervisees.
- Level 3i are referred to as "master supervisors" and are able to provide metasupervision themselves. Interestingly, in the EMDR system, one can theoretically start providing metasupervision and evaluating a

DOI: 10.4324/9781003214588-13

trainee-Consultant for accreditation as soon as one has qualified as a Consultant oneself. I would suggest that, ideally, metasupervision should not take be undertaken by newly qualified Consultants, at least for a year or two following Consultant accreditation.

Writers on clinical supervision frequently refer to the "four-stage competence model," sometimes attributed to Robinson (1974) and sometimes to Peyton (1998). These four stages are described by Bernard and Goodyear (2019) in the following way:

- Unconscious incompetence – "I don't know what I don't know"
- Conscious incompetence – "I know what I need to know"
- Conscious competence – "I know what to do and how"
- Unconscious competence – "My skills are so ingrained that I often do not have to think much about what to do when I work"

The fourth stage, "unconscious competence" reminds me, as an amateur trumpet player, of the fact that we develop "muscle memory" in which fast, complex behaviours become automatic because we could not possibly be consciously aware of the complexity of what we are doing. This may be wonderful and could make me a great trumpet player or therapist (potentially!). But it is not helpful to me as a supervisor because I cannot explain what I am doing if I am not conscious of it. Rather than unconscious competence, as supervisors, we need to develop "self-aware practice" (Bernard & Goodyear, 2019) so that we can explain to our supervisees what we are doing.

I recall, in my own training as a Clinical Psychologist, observing my very first placement supervisor seeing a client for their first session. After the session, I asked her why she was not following the comprehensive History Taking procedure that we had been taught in our training course. She replied that she had been doing this job for a long time and that she could suss out what was happening with a client fairly quickly and could therefore take some shortcuts. I have no doubt that she was right and with experience, I also do the same thing now. However, this was, I think, a case of unconscious competence, as she did not volunteer any guidance about how I could learn from this other than, "just wait until you're as experienced as me."

So far, this book has described the theory and skills required in order to supervise EMDR therapy. But what is the best way to train our budding EMDR Consultants in this role and how do we evaluate whether they are ready to become accredited as EMDR Consultants?

There are two main stages in the training of EMDR Consultants which are closely interlinked. The first of these is the four-day Consultants Training, which is one of the EMDR Europe requirements for accreditation as an EMDR Consultant. The second is the relationship that the trainee-Consultant has with their own supervisor in terms of their supervision-of-supervision and assessment of their supervisee's competence in relation to Consultant accreditation. These two stages are closely linked as the feedback from the Consultants Training will inform the supervisor regarding what progress needs to be made before their supervisee is ready for Consultant accreditation.

At what point should EMDR therapists commence training to be supervisors? Well, in one sense this training starts as soon as they begin to receive their own EMDR supervision after their Part 1 training. We learn by modelling and, just as many of us develop a parenting style based on our own experience of being parented, we model our supervision style on that of our own supervisors. Fleming (2012, p. 182) points out that clinicians should be learning about supervision as soon as they are being trained, "to provide the skills to trainees to enable them to play an active part in their own supervision" (p. 87).

Consultants training

Watkins and Wang (2014), in a review of the literature regarding supervisor training, conclude that the consensus is that the following are the most important to cover in the training of supervisors:

- Supervisor/supervisee roles and responsibilities
- Ethical/legal issues in supervision
- Models of supervision
- Assessment/evaluation in supervision
- Models of therapist development
- Establishing and maintaining the supervision alliance
- Supervision interventions/strategies
- Diversity in supervision
- Research about supervision

Not every accrediting organisation for psychological therapies requires that their accredited supervisors or consultants need to attend a formal training course. However, EMDR Europe specifies a 30-hour training course which, for example in the UK, is carried out over a four-day period. The format and content of this training is specified in Appendix 4.

Bernard and Goodyear (2019) describe the two broad areas of supervisor competence as:

"(a) knowledge and skills to provide the type of services their supervisees are providing
(b) knowledge and skills in supervision itself" (p. 266).

This is basically what our EMDR Consultants Training covers.

With regard to the first of these competencies, it might be assumed that an individual who has been accredited as an EMDR Practitioner would have been assessed by their own supervising Consultant as being fully cognisant of the EMDR protocol and skilled in its implementation. It is therefore surprising in Consultants Training how much "brushing up" of the basic Standard Protocol needs to happen for many of the participants. In the UK, the first of the four days of the training is devoted to this.

Many participants in the Consultants Training may have previous experience of supervising in other modalities and many will already have received some training in supervision. There are some similarities here with the situation when therapists start their basic training in EMDR therapy. Whilst their previous therapeutic experience will be useful and can be developed through their EMDR training, there will also need to be aspects of their way of working that have to be unlearned. In a basic EMDR training, for example, the necessity of "staying out of the way" when processing is occurring smoothly is difficult for some trainees to master. Similar difficulties of unlearning may arise during the Consultants Training. For example, an individual experienced in providing CBT supervision may use Socratic questioning in supervision rather than just providing some straight teaching where there is an apparent gap in the supervisee's knowledge.

There is some debate as to what point in their development individuals should attend the Consultants Training. Hawkins and McMahon (2020) suggest that one opinion is that "it might seem preferable that they receive training before they embark on giving any supervision, so that they have clarity about what they are providing and how they are going to function before they even start" (p. 160). However, they also point out that the limitation of this is that it leaves trainees with no experience on which to reflect and develop other than the experience of being supervised themselves. They suggest that some supervision training should be covered during the basic training of all therapists in order that they can become "better supervision consumers themselves" (Watkins & Wang, 2014, p. 182).

As stated in the EMDR Europe specification in Appendix 4, "it is strongly recommended that this training takes place at the beginning of a trainee Consultants Training." I would personally disagree with this. I believe that therapists should wait for at least a year after Practitioner accreditation before attending the Consultants Training. This would enable to establish themselves as competent therapists and start to get some experience in supervising others in EMDR. In this way, they are likely to learn more from the training when they receive it. In fact, the website of the EMDR Association UK, states, "It is recommended that consultants-in-training attend the Consultants Training after approximately 1–1.5 years of becoming accredited as an EMDR Practitioner to gain the optimum learning from attendance at the Consultants Training."

Unlike the basic EMDR training, the Consultants Training has an evaluative component. Trainees are assessed and the trainer produces a report which is passed on to the trainee's own supervisor. It is inevitable that trainees will feel that their "performance" is being assessed during the training, particularly in relation to the supervision role plays. As trainers, however, we are more interested in how trainees respond to feedback and their ability to learn from their own mistakes and those of others. The Consultant-in-training is also assessed at the training on the feedback that they provide to the "supervisor" about their supervision in the role play. If there is more work that needs to be done in a particular area, this can be done together with the trainee's own supervisor. In my own experience, the trainees who have not been able to reach a point where they are deemed to be competent by their supervisors are those who have been resistant to feedback and unable to appreciate where they need to develop and do more work on their own practice.

Supervision of supervision – "Metasupervision"

The second prong in the development of the EMDR Consultant is the supervision that they receive from their own Consultant supervisor. Bernard and Goodyear (2019) use the term "metasupervision" to describe the supervision of supervision, a term that I will adopt myself as it is much less unwieldy than "supervision of supervision."

Returning to Hawkins and Shohet's "Seven-Eyed model" (Hawkins & McMahon, 2020) (see Chapter 3), an additional fourth person has now been included – client, therapist, trainee-Consultant, Consultant – (Bernard & Goodyear, 2019) and instead of seven eyes we now have, perhaps, nine eyes. Occasionally, it can be more than that. One of my supervisees is an experienced EMDR Consultant. She wished to discuss problems that she was having with a supervisee who is, herself, an EMDR supervisor in relation to problems she was having with her own supervisee. In this case, the model would need to be expanded to eleven eyes!

On a couple of occasions, my own delivery of metasupervision has taken us to the Enabling function of supervision. In both cases, my supervisees, who were very competent EMDR Consultants, had supervisees who were high-status experts in their own fields but novices in relation to their EMDR practice and were both using EMDR beyond their level of competence. My supervisees both knew exactly what feedback they needed to give, but they needed to bolster the courage of their convictions. As their supervisor, I was able to remind them that, when it came to EMDR, *they* were the experts and could confidently provide the feedback that was necessary.

In Chapter 8, I reviewed the different media for delivering supervision. Most metasupervision takes place through verbal reports. However, the increased use of video conferencing, especially since the Covid-19 pandemic, has enhanced the possible ways of doing this. For example, one of my supervisees, a trainee-Consultant, was supervising several groups online and invited me to participate in some of these sessions. After each case was presented, I would add my comments about the particular case if I felt there was anything that my supervisee had not covered or if I thought there might be a more effective way of explaining something. We would then apportion the last 15 minutes of the session to just the supervisee and myself in order to provide her with some feedback about what had occurred in the session. An added bonus to this approach was that I did not need to see separate videos of her group supervision practice for purposes of Accreditation as this had already been observed live.

When I am supervising someone who is starting to provide supervision themselves, I use their own supervision sessions to teach them about the supervision process. So, often after we have finished discussing a particular case, I will ask the supervisee to reflect on what has just happened between us during that interaction. A story told in Chapter 3 is worth repeating here: When asking one of my supervisees for feedback about the case we had just discussed, she said, "I no longer feel like a useless therapist. I have realised that mum is not responding because she has her own unresolved trauma rather than because I am ineffective." I replied, "OK, so how did I help you with that?" She said, "by pointing this out and saying how you would feel in the same situation." This was helpful to us both. It helped me to know what I had done to help her with this particular case. But it also helped my supervisee to consciously reflect upon the process of supervision and to unpack the mechanism of how it can work.

Some EMDR Consultants find it difficult to accept that they are actually now Consultants and that they have the experience and expertise to work autonomously. There may be a tendency, during metasupervision, for the Consultant to ask their supervisor repeatedly whether they gave the right answer to their supervisee's SQs. Sometimes for the supervisor to just raise this as an issue during a review of the supervisory relationship can help the supervisee to realise that, "yes, I can stand on my own two feet now and I only need to bring my particularly tricky clients and supervisees to supervision." I have also used responses such as, "what answer do you think I would give?" or "why did you feel that you needed to ask me that?"

Accreditation as an EMDR consultant

The following are the current basic requirements for accreditation as an EMDR Europe Accredited Consultant:

- Minimum of three years experience as an EMDR Europe Accredited Practitioner
- Treated a broad range of clients of varying diagnoses and complexity
- A minimum of 400 EMDR sessions since becoming a Practitioner
- A minimum of 75 clients utilising EMDR since becoming a Practitioner
- Demonstrated competency in both provision of clinical supervision/consultation and of clinical work and have engaged in a minimum of 20 hours

of clinical supervision/consultation with an EMDR Europe Accredited Consultant
- Certificate of Competency from the EMDR Europe Consultants Training and had feedback from a Consultant Trainer regarding the applicant
- Minimum of 30 hours of EMDR-related Continuing Professional Development (CPD) and aware of current EMDR research
- Supervisor has witnessed a minimum of three videos, or in-vivo sessions meeting the required standard, of the applicant's professional practice of which one must be clinical, the second of them providing individual EMDR clinical supervision and the third of them providing group EMDR clinical supervision

In relation to the Certificate of Competency from the Consultants Training, this process starts after the Consultants Training when the Trainer completes a report relating to the trainee's performance during the training which is forwarded to both the trainee and their Consultant. This report will highlight the areas that the Trainer considers the trainee still needs to work on, and it is the responsibility of their own supervisor to ensure that these requirements have been covered. Once the Consultant is satisfied that the trainee is competent in these areas, they will inform the Trainer who will then issue the Certificate of Competency.

The EMDR Europe Competency-Based Framework also requires the supervising Consultant to comment on the applicant's skills in relation to the Standard Protocol as well as having knowledge and experience of the following protocols:

- EMDR, dissociation and Complex Post Traumatic Stress Disorder (C-PTSD)
- EMDR with phobias
- EMDR and clients with addictive behaviours
- EMDR and clients with pain
- EMDR protocols for acute trauma (Recent Events Protocol)
- EMDR and traumatic bereavement, grief, and mourning
- EMDR with depression
- EMDR with psychosis

To be honest, it would not be possible for every applicant to have direct experience in all these areas (e.g. psychosis) but they would certainly be expected to have some basic knowledge and awareness that these protocols exist and be able to point the supervisee in the direction of literature addressing these areas.

Specifically, in relation to their competence regarding supervision skills, the EMDR Europe Competency-Based Framework requires the supervisor to confirm the following:

- Basic approach and attitude towards supervisee's duties and responsibilities:
  - Development of a co-operative clinical supervision alliance with supervisees
  - Demonstration of a high level of professional attitude and competence
- Rapport building with Supervisees
  - Create a safe atmosphere within clinical supervision
  - Providing adequate and constructive feedback to supervisees
  - Developing an effective attunement and adequate coaching style
- Ability to transfer knowledge effectively to the theoretical framework of Adaptive Information Processing (AIP)
- Focuses on consultation on the following issues:
  - Practice of the Standard EMDR Protocol
  - Correct application of the protocol
  - Acknowledge recognition of other approaches or treatment plans and interventions
  - Demonstrate an ability to answer supervisees' questions effectively, considering the following:
    - Explore and clarify the question
    - Answer from a theoretical background
    - Answer on a practical level
    - Give specific hints and suggestions for specific case
    - Teach about differential diagnosis and/or alternative treatments
- Identify and effectively manage group processes

So, we are quite clear about our criteria. But how do we actually find out whether our supervisees fit these criteria? The published literature on clinical supervision appears to be sparse in this respect. There are plenty of published rating scales regarding supervisor competence (Watkins & Milne, 2014) but, at the end of the day, these are just lists. How do we ascertain whether our supervisees have developed the required competencies on our own list of criteria or those specified in any other list? Feeling somewhat gloomy whilst reaching this point in the writing of my book, I was cheered by finding the following which was reportedly posted on Albert Einstein's office wall: "Not everything that counts can be counted and not everything that can be counted counts."

Obviously, this is something we have already looked at in Chapter 6 in relation to the Evaluating component of supervision where it relates to the accreditation of Practitioners. As already said, the evaluation should, as much as possible, be a collaborative process between the supervisor and supervisee. The prospective EMDR Consultant, even more so than the prospective Practitioner, needs to be reflecting on their own practice because, as a supervisor, this is what they will be expecting their supervisees to do. By reflecting on their own work, how their supervisor responds to their work, and in particular, the discussions that arise from the supervisor witnessing their work (in vivo or by video), it would be hoped that both individuals in the supervision dyad will come to a moment of agreement that they are ready to become accredited.

Interestingly, my own experience is that the supervisees who are still far from ready for accreditation are those who lack insight and have great difficulty in reflecting on their own work in a critical but constructive way.

Sometimes it is during the Consultants Training that the realisation first occurs for the trainee-Consultant that either they need to do more work on themselves before becoming a Consultant or maybe it is just not for them. There is often feedback from the Consultants Training by trainees that they were put under too much pressure on the training. However, it must be acknowledged that being an EMDR Consultant is a pressurised job and, for example, includes teaching groups of supervisees who, may themselves, be high status in their profession and/or highly experienced in other therapies. Some trainees will recover from a bad experience on the Consultants Training and realise what work they need to do on themselves. Others, unfortunately, will realise that they are just not cut out for it.

It has to be accepted that there will be a small minority of EMDR therapists who will never reach a point where they are ready to become EMDR Consultants. Just because you are a good therapist does not mean that you can necessarily develop the skills to teach others to do the same.

Conclusion

Oh dear, that is a rather gloomy note to end the book on! As I said at the conclusion of Chapter 8, we cannot always find answers to every dilemma. However, what I have endeavoured to convey in this book is that, by reflecting on what we do and using some useful models, we can facilitate our supervisees in growing and developing as EMDR therapists, helping them to learn and feel supported whilst enlisting them in the task of evaluating their own practice.

In 2022, the year I finished writing this book, I also ran my own EMDR Consultants Training for the first time. What felt particularly important throughout this training was that we were able to reflect, in an open and honest way, on what we were doing. The trainees heard many stories from me about times I had got things wrong, which modelled for them a willingness to be open about their own vulnerabilities. Admittedly some trainees still found the training quite overwhelming and sometimes felt outside their Window of Tolerance. But, by constantly reflecting on what was happening as we learned together, we started to foster a collaborative way of understanding the EMDR supervision process. For me, this is what EMDR supervision is all about.

Bernard, J. M., & Goodyear, R. K. (2019). *Fundamentals of clinical supervision* (6th ed.). New York, NY: Pearson.

Fleming, I. (2012). Developments in supervisor training. In I. Fleming & L. Steen (Eds.), *Supervision and clinical psychology: Theory, practice and perspectives.* London, UK: Routledge.

Hawkins, P., & McMahon, A. (2020). *Supervision in the helping professions* (5th ed.). London: Open University Press.

Peyton, J. (1998). The learning cycle. In J. Peyton (Ed.), *Teaching and learning in medical practice* (pp. 13–19). Rickmansworth, UK: Manticore Europe Ltd.

Robinson, W. (1974). Conscious competency – The mark of a competent instructor. *The Personnel Journal, 53*, 538–539.

Stoltenberg, C. D., & McNeill, B. W. (2011). *IDM supervision: An integrative developmental model for supervising counselors and therapists* (3rd ed.). New York: Taylor and Francis.

Watkins, C. E., & Milne, D. (2014). *The Wiley international handbook of clinical supervision.* Chichester, UK: Wiley.

Watkins, C. E., & Wang, D. C. (2014). On the education of clinical supervisors. In C. E. Watkins & D. Milne (Eds.), *The Wiley international handbook of clinical supervision* (pp. 177–203). Chichester, UK: Wiley.

EMDR therapy consultation/supervision agreement

Jo Scott

Sample contract

The purpose of this agreement is to establish a clear understanding of the expectations of consultation/supervision.

I provide EMDR consultation and supervision to mental health professionals and therapists who have attended Parts 1–4 of their basic training in EMDR therapy and who wish to develop their skills in using this approach with children, adolescents, and adults. If required this can also include supporting EMDR therapists through the Accreditation process to become an EMDR Practitioner or EMDR Consultant. Consultation/supervision can be on an individual or group basis to mental health professionals from a variety of disciplines, who may be employed by NHS Trusts, other organisations, or who are in private practice. It can be provided "in person" or "online" and is usually on a 4–6 weekly basis.

Expectations and responsibilities of consultation/supervision

- EMDR consultation/supervision should be regarded as a specialist supervision, additional to any clinical or case management supervision required by the therapist's employer, organisation or core profession. As an EMDR Consultant, I do not hold clinical responsibility or liability for a supervisee's cases. As qualified and accredited mental health professionals they practice within their own professional codes of conduct and ethics and are accountable for their own practice.
- My role is to help the supervisee understand the technical aspects of integrating EMDR into the overall case conceptualisation and treatment plan and to enhance their understanding of the theoretical and practical application of EMDR. This will also involve exploring and identifying with them any possible risks or contra indicators for using EMDR at a particular time or in a particular situation, in order to enhance the service offered to the client and to ensure their welfare.

- The content of consultation/supervision will focus on the acquisition of knowledge, case conceptualisation and clinical skills within the EMDR therapy model and protocol. This will take the form of a variety of strategies, including constructive feedback, guidance and advice, reflective practice, and consideration of the therapeutic relationship and engagement issues.
- To keep the consultee/supervisee informed of trainings, research, and new developments within the EMDR and trauma-related field, including identification of ongoing CPD.
- The consultee/supervisee will be expected to complete and email a Supervision Case Presentation form to the Consultant/Supervisor **prior** to the supervision session in order to clarify the supervision question and enhance the learning experience.
- If undertaking the Accreditation process the consultee/supervisee will also be expected to submit video recordings of some therapeutic sessions, or arrange for the Consultant to directly observe their practice, as per the Accreditation criteria.

Confidentiality

- All professional and clinical issues discussed are confidential and are not to be discussed outside of the supervision session. The exceptions to this are to prevent the risk of serious harm, or if required to do so in compliance with the law.
- All cases or professionals discussed during supervision must be anonymised.
- Where video recording of sessions takes place this must be agreed with and have the informed, written consent of the client. Arrangements must also be made to destroy any recordings. The supervisee is responsible for ensuring this process is followed.

Practicalities/cancellation policy/fee

- Individual sessions will be either 30 or 60 minutes (as agreed)
- Group sessions will be 2 hours, with no more than 4 supervisees.
- Fees for supervision are £......... (as agreed) and to be paid by BACS (individual) or by invoice (monthly in arrears for organisations). <Supervisor's Name>......... Bank a/c: 1234567, Sortcode: 12-34-56
- Cancellation arrangements: 24 hours notice or full fee is payable

Consultee/supervisee's information

- Core profession and registered body:..
....

- Level of EMDR Training/qualifications and date obtained ....
....
....
- If wishing to work towards Accreditation the supervisee will need to supply copies of EMDR certificates (basic and C & A)
- **Contact details**:
- Name...
- Email.. Mobile:...........................

Signed.............................. EMDR Consultee/Supervisee. Date...........
Signed.............................. EMDR Consultant/Supervisor. Date...........

EMDR new supervisee checklist

Marian Tobin, 2022

Section 1: All new supervisees

- Core professional background; current registration/accreditation
- EMDR trainer – Ensure Europe accredited trainer
- Date of completion of EMDR Training – Certificate
- Accessibility needs to consider
- Current clinical work context – Statutory, voluntary, private
- CPD to date (EMDR and other mental health/trauma related)
- Working towards becoming an accredited practitioner

Section 2: Supervisee working towards EMDR practitioner accreditation

- Check all of Section 1 and the following:
- Name of previous EMDR-accredited clinical supervisor
- Number of cases, clinical activity to date, signed by the previous supervisor
- Clinical specialism
- C&A – Check child training, requires C&A consultant supervision
- CPD – EMDR and other mental health/trauma related
- Conference attendance
- EMDR activity; regional group, peer group, presentations, research, etc.
- Obtain evidence of clinical competence, current video material

Section 3: Supervisee working towards EMDR consultant accreditation

- Check Section 1 and the following:
- Date of EMDR practitioner accreditation – See certificate
- Current member of EMDR association?
- EMDR clinical activity to date, signed by the previous supervisor

- EMDR clinical supervision received to date, signed by the previous supervisor
- Provision of EMDR clinical supervision – Individual and group
- Ensure understanding regarding the status of their provision of supervision
- Specialism: Is supervision provided within the supervisee's area of knowledge/expertise?
- Obtain evidence of clinical competence, current video material
- C&A – Check child training, requires C&A consultant supervision
- Date of consultant training – See feedback list or Certificate if completed
- EMDR activity: Regional group, peer group, publications, presentations, etc.
- Understanding of EMDR accreditation process, competency framework
- CPD – EMDR and other mental health/trauma related
- EMDR National/European conference – Mandatory requirement for accreditation
- NB: Applications for accreditation as an EMDR practitioner or EMDR consultant must have client case list(s) signed by an accredited EMDR consultant

Section 4: New supervisee accredited practitioner/reaccreditation

- Core professional background; current registration/accreditation
- EMDR Trainer – Ensure EMDR Europe accredited trainer
- Date of completion of EMDR Training – See certificate
- Date of Practitioner accreditation – Check accreditation has not lapsed
- Current member of EMDR UK Association?
- Accessibility need(s) to consider
- Current clinical work context – Statutory, voluntary, private, etc.
- Name of previous EMDR consultant clinical supervisor
- Current hours of clinical practice
- EMDR specialism/clinical expertise
- EMDR activity: Research, SIG, Peer/Regional Groups, etc.
- CPD, EMDR Conference – Mandatory requirement for reaccreditation

Section 5: New supervisee accredited consultant/ reaccreditation

- Core professional background; current registration/accreditation
- EMDR trainer – Ensure Europe accredited trainer
- Date of completion of EMDR training – See certificate
- Date of EMDR Consultant accreditation – Check accreditation has not lapsed
- Current member of EMDR UK Association
- Accessibility need(s) to consider

- Name of previous EMDR consultant clinical supervisor, potential second reference
- Current hours of EMDR clinical practice
- Current provision of EMDR clinical supervision – Individual/group
- EMDR specialism/clinical expertise
- EMDR Activity: Research, SIG, Peer/Regional Groups, etc.
- CPD – EMDR and other mental health/trauma related
- EMDR National/European Conference – Mandatory requirement for reaccreditation
- EMDR consultants day – Mandatory requirement for reaccreditation

EMDR Europe competency framework

The competency framework agreed by EMDR Europe for accreditation as an EMDR Practitioner is shown as follows.

Part A

Supervisee demonstrates a grounded understanding of the theoretical basis of EMDR and the Adaptive Information Processing (AIP) Model and is able to convey this effectively to clients in providing a treatment overview.

Part B: The basic eight-phase protocol

1. History taking

The supervisee is able to take an appropriate general history from the client incorporating the following elements:

- Obtains a history of the origins of the disorder informed by the AIP model, including dysfunctional behaviour and symptoms.
- Determines if the client is appropriate for EMDR selection. Identifies "red flags" including screening for Dissociative Disorders.
- Is able to identify appropriate safety factors including the use (where appropriate) of the Dissociative Experience Scale II (DES), Risk Assessment, Life Constraints, Ego Strength, and the availability of support structures.
- Demonstrates an ability to conceptualise the case using the AIP model.
- Clarifies the client's desired state following therapeutic intervention.
- Ensures that the client is able to deal effectively with high levels of physical and emotional disturbance.
- Determines appropriate target selection and target sequencing in relation to past, present, and future.
- In cases of multiple targets, is able to prioritise or cluster.
- Identifies a "touchstone" event that relates to the client's issue.

2. Preparation

The supervisee is able to establish an effective therapeutic relationship in conformance with National or Professional standards and Code of Conduct:

- Obtains informed consent from clients.
- Tests Bilateral Stimulation (BLS) with clients.
- Teaches and checks client's ability to self-regulate, including the use of safe/secure place and resource installation.
- Makes clients aware of the "Stop" signal.
- Demonstrates effective ability to address client concerns, fears, queries or anxieties.
- Using effective metaphors.

3. Assessment

During the "Assessment Phase," the supervisee determines the components of the target memory and establishes baseline measures for the client's reactions to the process:

- Selects target image and worst aspect.
- Identifies the negative and positive cognitions.
- Establishes negative cognitions that reflect a currently held, negative self-referencing belief that is irrational, generalisable, and has affect resonance that accurately focuses upon the target issue.
- Ensures cognitions are within the same domain/matched category.
- When necessary the supervisee effectively helps the client to identify pertinent NCs and PCs.
- Uses the Validity of Cognition (VOC) scale at an emotional level, and in direct relation to the target.
- Identifies emotions generated from the target issue or event.
- Demonstrates consistent use of the Subjective Units of Disturbance (SUDs) scale to evaluate the total disturbance.
- Identifies body sensations and location.

4. Desensitisation

During the "Desensitisation Phase," the supervisee processes the dysfunctional material stored in all channels associated with the target event and any ancillary channels:

- Reminds clients to "just notice" whatever comes up during processing, while encouraging client not to disregard any information that might be generated.

- Explains that changes during processing can relate to images, sounds, cognitions, emotions, and physical sensations.
- Demonstrates competency in the provision of Bilateral Stimulation (BLS), emphasising the importance of eye movements.
- Uses appropriate post-set interventions, and shows evidence of "staying out of the way" as much as possible.
- Reassures client verbally and non-verbally during each set.
- Maintains momentum throughout the desensitisation stage with minimal intervention where possible.
- Returns to target when appropriate.
- When processing becomes blocked, uses appropriate interventions including alteration in Bilateral Simulation and/or the use of Cognitive Interweaves. (Please specify examples of effective Cognitive Interweaves used during the Desensitisation Phase when processing has become blocked.)
- Effectively manages heightened levels of client affect using both accelerating and de-accelerating interventions.

5. Installation

During the "Installation Phase," the supervisee concentrates primarily upon the full integration of a positive self-assessment with the targeted information:

- Enhances the Positive Cognition (PC) linked specifically with the target issue or event.
- Checks Positive Cognition for both applicability and current validity, ensuring the PC chosen is the most meaningful to the client.
- Uses the Validity of Cognition (VOC) scale to evaluate the Positive Cognition.
- Addresses any blocks during the Installation Phase.
- If new material emerges, supervisee effectively returns to the most appropriate phase of the EMDR Protocol or uses the "Incomplete Session."

6. Body scan

During the "Body Scan Phase," the supervisee considers the link between the client's original memory/event and the discernible physical resonance that this may generate:

- The supervisee enables clients to hold both the memory/event and the Positive Cognition in mind while mentally scanning their entire body to

identify any lingering tension, tightness or unusual sensation, and applies Bilateral Stimulation (BLS).
- The supervisee is prepared for further material to surface and to respond accordingly, by either returning to the most appropriate phase of the EMDR Protocol or using the "Incomplete Session."

7. Closure

The supervisee should consistently close a session with proper instruction, leaving the client in a positive frame of mind and able to return safely home:

- Allows time for closure.
- Uses the debrief.
- Effectively uses the "Incomplete Session."
- Uses appropriate containment exercises and safety assessment.
- Encourages clients to maintain a log between sessions.

8. Re-evaluation of previous session

During the "Re-evaluation Phase," the supervisee consistently assesses how well the previously targeted material has been resolved and determines if new processing is necessary. The supervisee actively integrates the targeting session within an overall treatment plan:

- Returns to previous targets.
- Identifies evidence of client re-adjustment.
- Determines whether the individual target has been resolved.
- Identifies any other material that has been activated and needs addressing.
- Ensures that all necessary targets have been processed in relation to the past, present and future.
- Uses when necessary a "Future/Positive Template."
- Ensures that client has readjusted appropriately to their social system.
- Effectively ends client's therapy.

Part C

- Supervisee demonstrates an understanding of PTSD and traumatology.
- Supervisee demonstrates an understanding of the use of EMDR either as part of a comprehensive therapy intervention or as a means of symptom reduction.
- Supervisee demonstrates experience in applying the standard EMDR protocol and procedures to special situations and clinical problems, including recent events, phobias, excessive grief, and somatic disorders.

EMDR Europe consultant's training course

The following represents the minimum requirements for an EMDR consultants training course. Trainers may add to any part of the course.

Eligibility

All candidates for training must provide one letter of recommendation from their EMDR consultant stating that they are ready to undertake training, plus a letter of support from their national association.

All candidates must have been accredited as an EMDR practitioner for at least one year prior to commencing this training.

Training should be open to any practitioner who meets the above requirement.

It is strongly recommended that this training takes place at the beginning of a trainee consultants training.

Outline of the course

1 **Review of the Accreditation Process and Competency Framework (2 hours)**
   Review of the EMDR Europe competency framework for both practitioner and consultant. Participants should be assessed on their understanding of the guidelines and the accreditation process from both a national and EMDR Europe perspective. (It is advisable to have a representative from the national association present during this part of the training.)

2 **Theory review (6 hours)**
   The following areas should be covered through teaching and practical exercises:

   - Psychotrauma
   - The neurobiology of trauma
   - Review of the AIP Model and EMDR Protocol

- Case conceptualisation
- Knowledge of evidence base
- Identify knowledge required in addition to that of a practitioner
- The importance of the therapeutic relationship in EMDR treatment
- Overview of scripted protocols, e.g.,

  - EMDR, dissociation and complex post-traumatic stress disorder (C-PTSD)
  - EMDR with phobias
  - EMDR and clients with addictive behaviours
  - EMDR and clients with pain
  - EMDR protocols for acute trauma (Recent Events Protocol)
  - EMDR and traumatic bereavement, grief, and mourning

3 **Teaching the consultation process (6 hours)**

- Definitions of consultation
- Different models of consultation and clinical supervision
- Difference between individual and group supervision
- The functions of supervision
- Supervisors' styles
- How EMDR supervision differs from generic supervision
- Roles of EMDR consultant as (i) educator and (ii) evaluator
- EMDR consultant's gate-keeping responsibilities for EMDR accreditation
- Managing the consultant/supervisee relationship
- Managing supervisees who do not meet EMDR Europe competence requirements
- Recognising supervisee own resistance, and trauma and affect phobia

4 **Assessing competence through live practice/video (10 hours)**
Training should include live consultation of the consultant-in-training supervising a course participant's case material, and/or live consultation of consultant-in-training's supervision video.

The consultant-in-training should also be assessed on their ability to transfer knowledge effectively to the supervisee on any of the above topics related to EMDR, AIP and trauma. This should be done by live consultation, or by role play.

5 **Evaluation (6 hours)**
Participants should be evaluated on all areas of knowledge and practice by the trainer, outlining both the consultant-in-training's strengths and weaknesses. This evaluation will form part of the consultant-in-training's final accreditation evaluation. The procedure for doing this must be negotiated with the national association.

6 **Duration of Training**
Minimum of 30 hours

7   Consultant trainer

The consultant training course should only be run by an EMDR Europe Senior Trainer. This condition may be waived for a new association who do not yet have a senior Trainer but only with the agreement of the standards committee. The trainer should have the support of the national association.

Approved 30.10.2016

Index

Note: Locators in *italics* represent figures and **bold** indicate tables in the text.

For Product Safety Concerns and Information please contact our EU
representative GPSR@taylorandfrancis.com Taylor & Francis Verlag GmbH,
Kaufingerstraße 24, 80331 München, Germany

Printed and bound by CPI Group (UK) Ltd, Croydon, CR0 4YY

08/06/2025
01896986-0019